Homelessness and Social Work

Drawing on intersectional theorising, *Homelessness and Social Work* highlights the diversities and complexities of homelessness and social work research, policy and practice. It invites social work students, practitioners, policy makers and academics to re-examine the subject by exploring how homelessness and social work are constituted through intersecting and unequal power relations.

The causes of homelessness are frequently associated with individualist explanations, without examining the broader political and intersecting social inequalities that shape how social problems such as homelessness are constructed and responded to by social workers. In reflecting on factors such as Indigeneity, race, ethnicity, gender, class, age, sexuality, ability and other markers of identity the author seeks to:

- construct a new intersectional framework for understanding social work and homelessness;
- provide a critical analysis of social work responses to homelessness;
- challenge how homelessness is represented in social work research, social policy and social work practice; and
- incorporate the stories of people experiencing homelessness.

The book will be of interest to undergraduate and higher research degree students in the fields of intersectionality, homelessness, sociology, public policy and social work.

Carole Zufferey is a senior lecturer at the School of Psychology, Social Work and Social Policy, University of South Australia. She has a social work background. Prior to entering academia, she practised in the fields of community welfare, child protection and youth justice in remote Western Australia; aged care and disability in London, UK; and mental health and homelessness in Adelaide, South Australia. She has published numerous journal articles and book chapters on social work, homelessness and intersectionality. Her recent research projects include exploring lived experiences of and diverse perspectives on home and homelessness, and the impact of domestic violence on women's citizenship, including on their mental health, housing, employment and social participation.

Routledge Advances in Social Work

New titles

Analysing Social Work Communication
Discourse in practice
*Edited by Christopher Hall, Kirsi Juhila, Maureen Matarese
and Carolus van Nijnatten*

Feminisms in Social Work Research
Promise and possibilities for justice-based knowledge
Edited by Stéphanie Wahab, Ben Anderson-Nathe and Christina Gringeri

Chronic Illness, Vulnerability and Social Work
Autoimmunity and the contemporary disease experience
Liz Walker and Elizabeth Price

Social Work in a Global Context
Issues and challenges
Edited by George Palattiyil, Dina Sidhva and Mono Chakrabarti

Contemporary Feminisms in Social Work Practice
Edited by Nicole Moulding and Sarah Wendt

Domestic Violence Perpetrators
Evidence-informed responses
John Devaney and Anne Lazenbatt

Transnational Social Work and Social Welfare
Challenges for the social work profession
*Edited by Beatrix Schwarzer, Ursula Kämmerer-Rütten,
Alexandra Schleyer-Lindemann and Yafang Wang*

The Ecosocial Transition of Societies
The contribution of social work and social policy
Edited by Aila-Leena Matthies and Kati Närhi

Responsibilization at the Margins of Welfare Services
Edited by Kirsi Juhila, Suvi Raitakari and Christopher Hall

Forthcoming titles

Homelessness and Social Work
An intersectional approach
Carole Zufferey

Supporting Care Leavers' Educational Transitions
Jennifer Driscoll

Homelessness and Social Work

An intersectional approach

Carole Zufferey

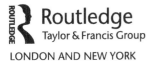

Routledge
Taylor & Francis Group

LONDON AND NEW YORK

First published 2017 by Routledge

2 Park Square, Milton Park, Abingdon, Oxfordshire OX14 4RN
52 Vanderbilt Avenue, New York, NY 10017

Routledge is an imprint of the Taylor & Francis Group, an informa business

First issued in paperback 2018

British Library Cataloguing in Publication Data
A catalogue record for this book is available from the British Library

Library of Congress Cataloguing in Publication Data
A catalog record for this book has been requested.

ISBN: 978-1-138-85877-0 (hbk)
ISBN: 978-0-367-15219-2 (pbk)

Typeset in Times New Roman
by Out of House Publishing

Contents

Acknowledgements

This book draws on different research projects that I have completed dating back to 2001. Thank you to all the research participants involved in these projects. This includes people who experienced homelessness, social workers and community informants who were interviewed for the various studies referred to in this book.

Thank you to Routledge for their interest in this work and the University of South Australia for their support to complete this book.

Many people have contributed to this book. First, I would like to thank Dr Christopher Horsell, for his ongoing commentary on the development of the book, for contributing a reflexive case study for Chapter 5 and his ongoing support in life.

As well, many thanks to Dr Margaret Rowntree for her editorial and conceptual support, her contribution to the book synopsis and her insightful feedback on the content, structure and writing of this book.

I would like to thank Professor Donna Chung, who supervised me in my MSW and PhD research studies, for her ongoing support and mentorship over the last 15 years. Our inspiring conversations have helped to shape my thinking about gender, domestic violence, homelessness, social work and intersectionality.

Finally, I would like to thank Associate Professor Adrian Vicary for his insights on academic scholarship during the writing of my PhD thesis.

Thanks also to my colleagues, Dr Nilan Yu and Dr Shepard Masocha, for our ongoing conversations about the complexities of writing and thinking about race and racism, that helped me think beyond gendered relations and homelessness.

I dedicate this book to my son Andre.

1   Introduction

Homelessness is a topical issue generating substantial attention in Western countries. While there is considerable research on the subject, little has been written on intersectional social work approaches to homelessness. Homelessness is complex and diverse because it intersects with other social issues (such as gendered violence), and with multiple social markers that include gender, class, race, sexuality and ability. As well, understandings of both homelessness and social work are contested, and vary according to different countries and organisational contexts. Complicating matters further, both service users and providers are constituted by the complex interplay of these multiple social locations.

This book is the first to promote an intersectional approach for social workers addressing homelessness. It builds upon my recent chapters in edited books on feminist research and practice in social work (see Wahab *et al.*, 2015; Wendt and Moulding, 2016). I use a critical and social constructionist epistemology, to explore how homelessness and social work are constituted through intersecting and unequal power relations. Following the work of social work scholars Hulko (2015) and Murphy *et al.* (2009), I advocate for adopting an intersectional approach that incorporates reflections on both oppression and privilege. This project is not situated exclusively within a particular school of thought, such as a structural or post-structural feminism. My intersectional approach in this book combines and draws on both critical/structural and post-structural ideas and theoretical perspectives. I argue that engaging with both structural and post-structural thought enables a more comprehensive and complex analysis of the topic of homelessness. It is this multi-faceted analysis that can then assist social workers to attend to the diversities of homelessness, and to advocate for 'the homeless' using new knowledge, research methods and practices. I also draw on Winker and Degele's (2011) conceptualisation of intersectionality that highlights the intersection of social structures, institutionalised organisational practices, multiple identities, cultural symbols and discursive representations of social problems. My intersectional social work approach has been developed through researching the perspectives of people from diverse social locations who experience homelessness, and of social workers who work with them, linking their subjective experiences (the micro), with social structures and institutionalised practices (the mezzo and the macro).

My argument in this book is that intersectionality provides a new way of understanding homelessness and social work research, social policy and social work practice. I examine how homelessness is constituted through unequal and intersecting power relations in social processes and social identity categorisations (or social locations), related to Indigeneity, race, ethnicity, gender, class, age, sexuality, ability and other markers of identity. I also explore how social work and responses to homelessness are constituted, by reflecting on social workers' own positions of power and often invisible privileges (and oppressions). The social locations of social workers can relate to white race privilege, class, ability, being employed, educated or other markers of privileged identities, as well as unequal power relations in client–worker relationships and social work processes. Therefore, in this book I highlight the intersecting diversities and complexities of homelessness and social work research, policy and practice, by proposing an intersectional social work approach.

The complexities of intersectionality

The scope of intersectionality is contested and debated. Intersectional theorists have particularly drawn upon structuralist approaches to identity (or subjectivity) 'as informed by various systems of oppression relating to race, class, gender and sexuality' (McKibbin *et al.*, 2015, p. 99). Intersectionality is a study of intersections between different systems of discrimination and *a way of thinking* about multiple identities and interconnected oppressions/ privileges in both men and women's lives (Crenshaw, 1991; Mehrotra, 2010; Hulko, 2015). This approach highlights multi-dimensional intersections related to for example, gender, sexuality, race/skin colour, ethnicity, nation/ state, class, culture, ability, age, sedentariness, origin, wealth, religion, geographical locations and social development (Lutz *et al.*, 2011). However, there is slippage 'between structuralist and post-structuralist ontologies' in intersectional literature, causing some confusion about 'the relationship between post-structuralist feminism, postcolonial feminism and intersectionality' (McKibbin *et al.*, 2015, p. 100). Social work and feminist scholars such as Murphy *et al.* (2009) and McKibbin *et al.* (2015) take different epistemological positions towards intersectionality. Unlike Murphy *et al.*'s (2009) more structuralist approach, McKibbin *et al.* (2015, p. 101) argue for a post-structural orientation to intersectionality as a 'discourse'. They argue that post-structural feminist orientations open up more possibilities for analyses of social problems, including men's violence against women. However, in this book, I argue that both theoretical perspectives can contribute to social work approaches to homelessness, depending on the purpose of the political project. These contestations, including Lykke's (2010) 'post-constructionist' theorising of intersectionality, are further discussed in the next chapter.

Whilst acknowledging the critiques of intersectionality as providing a 'handy catchall phrase' (Phoenix and Pattynama, 2006, p. 187), I argue that an intersectional approach can contribute to new ways of reflecting on homelessness and social work. Intersectionality is useful for analysing the various ways in which different social divisions and power relations are enmeshed and constructed. It allows for a more complex, fluid, multilayered analysis of diverse social identities (or subjectivities) and social locations, and for a more thorough reflexive exploration of how social processes and relationships intersect and continue to uphold social inequalities (Damant *et al.*, 2008; Lykke, 2010). Intersectionality can provide a new social work approach that makes visible the 'multiple positioning that constitutes everyday life and the power relations' (Phoenix and Pattynama, 2006, p. 187), and contributes to shaping the complexities of social work and homelessness. It can also be a powerful tool for social workers to examine their own privileges (and oppressions).

Similar to Hulko's (2009, p. 52) vision for intersectionality, my hope for this book is that it will help social workers and social work students 'appreciate that they can be both oppressors and the oppressed at the same time'. For example, we can be aware of our 'marginal social status' (such as Aboriginal ancestry or ethno-cultural background), yet not have considered our 'social-class position' (Hulko, 2009, p. 52). However, it is also important to note that some intersectional oppressions/privileges can change over time and in different social contexts. Thus, we cannot homogenise the ways political projects affect different people (Yuval Davis, 2006; 2012). In regards to homelessness, this approach would involve not sliding into essentialism, such as pointing out the characteristics of 'the homeless', and reductionism, such as arguing that there is one cause of homelessness.

In this book, I aim to rethink how the 'problem' of homelessness is understood and addressed by social workers. I am not arguing that social work is the only discipline that has a claim to the issue, as many different professions are involved in responding to homelessness. However, this book draws on my own research and expertise, which is in the field of social work and homelessness. I come to this work with experience as a social work practitioner in multi-disciplinary and multi-cultural teams in Australia and the UK that included responding to the diversity of homelessness and other social issues, such as the wellbeing and protection of children, disability, ageing and mental health. For over 15 years I have been researching homelessness and social work, particularly in the Australian context. More recently, I have been engaged in exploring the relevance of intersectionality to social work and homelessness (Zufferey, 2009; 2015; 2016b).

There is one book on intersectionality and social work (Murphy *et al.*, 2009) but no previous books have combined a focus on intersectionality, social work and homelessness. The assumptions that underpin intersectionality are consistent with those of social work, as they are about social change, building coalitions and working to upholding social justice and human rights.

Intersectional analyses are useful in the fields of homelessness and social work by:

- placing the lived experiences of marginalised groups at the centre of the development of theory and research (Hulko, 2015), such as making visible the diverse perspectives of people experiencing homelessness;
- being 'majority inclusive' and thus, enabling a reflection on constructions of privilege and privileging practices (Christensen and Jensen, 2012), such as social workers' reflecting on our own privileges (Hulko, 2015);
- exploring the complexities of individual and group identities, while highlighting the ways in which diversity within groups is often ignored and/ or homogenised (Dhamoon, 2011), including by not homogenising 'the homeless experience';
- demonstrating how social inequality and oppression manifest in interconnected domains of power relations (Thornton Dill and Zambrana, 2009; Thornton Dill and Kohlman, 2012), including power relations relevant to social workers responding to people experiencing homelessness; and
- promoting social justice and social change, such as through social work advocacy, research, policy, practice and education (Murphy *et al.*, 2009).

In this book I draw on these theoretical and methodological complexities, which distinguishes it from other work in the fields of social work and homelessness.

The complexities of homelessness

Homelessness is also a contested concept. Homelessness is frequently constructed as 'rough sleeping' or 'houselessness'. These housing-based definitions of homelessness assume that 'houselessness' is the problem and housing is the solution (Tomas and Dittmar, 1995; Zufferey, 2016a). Such normative definitions and understandings of homelessness in Western countries often fail to incorporate multiple and diverse perspectives of home and homelessness (Zufferey, 2016a; 2016b). Also, the relevance of Western definitions of homelessness for developing countries has been questioned (Tipple and Speak, 2009). Whilst it is important for social workers to advocate for access to safe and affordable housing, it is also important to make visible alternative perspectives and experiences of homelessness. Homelessness is inextricably connected to intersecting sites of disadvantage and inequality, which include global and local issues, Western global domination, class elitism, unequal gender and power relations, homophobia and white race privilege. Intersectional analyses enable social work researchers, policy makers and practitioners to examine how these diverse inequalities intersect in social processes and contribute to shaping the experiences and subjectivities of men and women who are defined as homeless.

Moreover, power relations constitute social work processes that can reproduce social inequalities, so it is also important to research the perspectives of both people who experience homelessness, and social workers who respond to homelessness. For example, social work research, policy and educational practices often involve defining and homogenising 'marginalised' or 'vulnerable' population groups. Likewise, social work practices tend to construct 'clients' who experience homelessness as the homogenous 'other' who are in 'need' of social work 'intervention' (Zufferey and Kerr, 2004). As well, social-policy-making processes constitute social 'problems' (such as homelessness) in particular ways (Bacchi, 2009). Intersectional analyses can make these social processes and multiple and intersecting power inequalities more visible, expanding on how social workers engage with socially constructed problems such as homelessness.

Whilst homelessness is a complex and emerging area of research for social workers, it is not a new phenomenon. Homelessness has long been a multidimensional human rights issue. The United Nations (UN) General Assembly adopted the Universal Declaration of Human Rights in 1948 (Article 25), which states that everyone has the right to a standard of living that is adequate for their health and wellbeing, including access to food, clothing, housing and medical care. Worldwide, there are over 100 million people without shelter; at least 1.6 billion people who lack adequate housing, and one in four people who live in housing situations that can affect their health and safety (Habitat, 2015), many of whom are women and children. Global definitions of homelessness have tended to focus on people being literally homeless (without shelter), with few possessions, 'sleeping in the streets, in doorways or on piers, or in any other space, on a more or less random basis'.[1] More recently, in 2016, the special United Nations Rapporteur on the Right to Adequate Housing, Leilani Farha, provided a three-dimensional definition of homelessness anchored in human rights and social inequality. She suggests that the first definitional dimension highlights 'the absence of home in terms of both its physical structure and its social aspects'; the second dimension focuses on 'systemic discrimination and social exclusion'; and the third dimension acknowledges that people are 'resilient in the struggle for survival and dignity and potential agents of change as rights holders' (UNHR, 2016, p. 1). Consistent with the United Nations, I also posit that homelessness is connected to systemic and structural patterns of discrimination that disproportionately affect people on the basis of gender, age, cultural background, ability, poverty, sexuality, migration and refugee status, each in different ways (UNHR, 2016). Policy definitions of homelessness are examined in further depth in Chapter Four.

Intersectional theorising acknowledges how home and homelessness is experienced differently, depending on one's social power, privilege and social location/s. In this book I reflect on the complexities of intersectionality, social work and homelessness by drawing on a number of research projects, including my own, and by examining social work literature on research, policy and practice responses to the issue. However, social work itself has been criticised for being ethnocentric, influenced by white, Western and middle-class discourses that are embodied and performed by social workers in their professional practices. As a white, Western, middle-class social work educator and practitioner, I continually question how my own gender, class and whiteness shapes my worldview, grants me particular privileges and informs my own research and practice in the area of homelessness (Zufferey, 2013). I have found intersectionality to be most useful for reflecting on the complex power dynamics in my responses to homelessness. I suggest that this reflexivity can, likewise, enable other social workers to explore how responses to homelessness are constituted by unequal institutionalised practices, and intersecting social locations and power relations. This argument is developed further in Chapter 5.

The complexities of social work

There are a number of claims made in social work literature to define the aims and purpose of the 'profession'. Globally, a set of universal values and ethics has been constructed to describe 'ideal' types of social work (Gibelman, 1999; McKay and Zufferey, 2015). Social work scholar Dunk-West (2013, p. 13) argues that whilst national policies and contemporary social and economic contexts frame social work, the profession's identity is clear because social workers across the world share similar professional values and theory bases. These ethics involve addressing inequalities and social justice in diverse settings, in order to promote the rights of disadvantaged people. However, social work professional identity and ethical practice is contested. For example, Payne (2014) notes that social work is socially constructed and 'clients', 'social workers' and the process called 'social work' are socially and historically embedded within organisational contexts and institutional regimes of power that change over time and in different contexts. As Shardlow (2009, p. 37) observes, while codes of ethics are universal ideals that can offer generalised and definitive answers, ethical practice is actually 'complex, messy and imprecise'. That is, social workers can resist social injustices, while at the same time, contribute to maintaining them. For example, in his analysis of policy and media discourses about constructions of asylum seekers, Masocha (2015, p. 7) explored the dominance of xenoracism, which is 'a rhetorically managed type of prejudice aimed at the discrimination, exclusion and marginalisation of asylum seekers', and found that these discourses also shape social worker's constructions of asylum seeker's subjectivities.

Social work authors such as Dominelli (2002) and Payne (2014) argue that social work is constructed through three dominant approaches: the 'therapeutic helping' or reflexive-therapeutic position; the emancipatory or socialist-collectivist position, and the individualist-reformist or maintenance position. Consistent with the social justice focus of the emancipatory social work approach, scholars in other disciplines such as women's studies and political science point to the value of radical and disruptive aspects of intersectionality in unsettling 'oppressive vehicles of power' (Dhamoon, 2011, p. 230; May, 2015). Likewise, social work author Hulko (2009, p. 53) acknowledges that systems of oppression and privilege intersect within historically and culturally situated social contexts that promote racism, heterosexism and ageism. Drawing on a range of multidisciplinary scholars, I argue that an intersectional social work approach to homelessness can combine different epistemological positions and intersect individual/structural, personal/political and micro/macro approaches, in ways that contribute to the social justice project of social work. A reflexive, intersectional approach can also highlight how social workers contribute to maintaining unequal power relations, which opens up possibilities for focusing on new areas for social work advocacy.

My thinking for this book emerged from my doctoral research in which I critically examined how homelessness (and service provision) is socially constructed in the public domain (as represented in the Australian print media), and how these constructions influenced research, social policy and social work responses to homelessness (Zufferey and Chung, 2006; Zufferey, 2007). I have previously argued that three particular points are important in understanding social work responses to homelessness (see Zufferey, 2008). First, social work and social policy approaches to homelessness are culturally and historically situated within broader Western individualist discourses about social problems. Second, welfare reforms of increasingly conservative Western governments that emphasise individual self-interest and moral responsibility shape public discourses, research, policy and practice responses to homelessness. For example, in Canada, the US, the UK, Australia and Scandinavia, 'welfare to work' policies introduced for welfare recipients, such as single parent families that oblige sole parents to look for work, are morally driven (Pulkingham *et al.*, 2010). Social workers who work in employment services become part of this monitoring system, and being homeless does not exempt people from the work activity test or compliance requirements, despite inherent difficulties in accessing and maintaining work. Third, socio-political agendas such as neoliberalism shape organisational contexts, and social work practice can be defined and constrained within these organisational settings (see also Gordon and Zufferey, 2013). Social workers perform their work within institutionalised practices and organisational discourses that constitute their responses to homelessness, and reflect dominant power relations between service providers and service users (Zufferey, 2008, p. 358).

This book is committed to making visible the perspectives of men and women with diverse experiences of homelessness, as well as reflecting on power relations in social work approaches to addressing the issue. However, it is also important to not fix 'homeless' and 'homed' identities, and to understand that intersecting social identities and locations are fluid and changing, and are temporally and spatially contingent on context. That is, even social workers can become homeless. As Emslie (2011) observes, youth housing workers in

Australia are paid wages so low that they too experience housing affordability stress and are at risk of, or living in, conditions defined as 'homeless'.

The lived experiences of people who may or may not define themselves as 'homeless' are diverse, multiple and shift across time and place. Intersectional social work approaches offer multiple 'entry point/s for social change efforts' and 'reflect the socially constructed nature of reality' (Hulko, 2009, p. 53). These approaches provide diverse opportunities to advocate for a more socially just social work. Therefore, I argue that intersectional theorising reso-nates with the complexities of homelessness and social work, consistent with the aims of this book, namely:

1   To construct a new intersectional approach for understanding social work and homelessness.
2   To provide a critical analysis of unequal power relations in social work responses to homelessness.
3   To challenge how homelessness is represented and responded to in social work research, social policy and social work practice.

To illustrate, in this book I present my own intersectional research on the diverse perspectives and identifications with home/s and homelessness (Chapter 3); on social workers' perspectives about their experiences of responding to homelessness (Chapter 5), and research that incorporates the diverse voices of people experiencing homelessness (Chapter 6).

Overview of book

This book has seven chapters. In this introductory chapter I have introduced the main concepts and arguments covered in this book, including definitions and debates in the fields of intersectionality, homelessness and social work. I have emphasised the complexities of intersectionality, homelessness and social work. I have also put forward my position that an intersectional approach can highlight unequal power relations that constitute homelessness and social work responses to it.

Chapter 2 examines literature on intersectionality in more depth. In this chapter I note that intersectional approaches can transcend individual and structural debates in homelessness and social work literature. I discuss debates about intersectionality within multidisciplinary literature, including social work, sociology, political science and women and gender studies, and present critiques of it. In this chapter I make the case that multidisciplinary intersectional theorising can be integrated into an intersectional social work approach to homelessness.

Chapter 3 analyses social work research on homelessness (and related social problems such as intimate partner violence) and intersectionality. In this chapter I critically examine research literature in the field of social work and homelessness, including how this literature does (or does not) draw on intersectionality. By presenting some of my own 'intersectional-type' research, I demonstrate how intersectionality in the fields of social work and homelessness can be valuable in informing these current bodies of research knowledge.

Chapter 4, on social policy and homelessness, examines intersectional policy analysis approaches in literature. In this chapter I discuss Hankivsky's (2012) Intersectionality-Based Policy Analysis (IBPA), and Bacchi's (2009) 'What's the problem represented to be?' (WPR) policy analysis frameworks. Then, I analyse definitions of homelessness in legislation, policy and service initiatives such as 'Housing First' in the USA, UK, Australia, New Zealand and the European Union. I argue that intersectional policy development and analysis can contribute to new understandings of policy approaches to homelessness, and social work research.

Chapter 5 focuses on 'frontline' service delivery and social work practice responses to homelessness. In this chapter I demonstrate how an intersectional approach provides further insights into how social workers can promote practices aligned with their commitments to challenging social injustice and human rights violations (Murphy *et al.*, 2009). To illustrate that an intersectional approach can broaden social workers' analyses and responses to homelessness, I present findings from my research interviews with social work managers, policy workers and frontline practitioners in Australia. I argue that social workers embody intersecting power relations, and that gendered, racialised and classed social locations constitute their understandings of social work, and responses to homelessness. In the spirit of the reflexivity of my intersectional social work approach to homelessness, I provide personal commentary and a case study. The first reflection comprises my own personal and professional engagement with homelessness and intersectionality. The second case study was constructed by Dr Chris Horsell, reflecting on when he was employed in the field of men's homelessness, working with a transgender client who identified as a woman. In this chapter I show how an intersectional social work approach can subvert dominant practices, expand social work advocacy, and make visible privilege and diverse power inequalities.

Chapter 6 highlights research and literature on lived experiences of homelessness. In this chapter, I present a diversity of perspectives and experiences of people, who are defined as 'homeless' by policy makers and service providers, but who do not necessarily define themselves as such. I commence the chapter by presenting my original research on 'everyday' lived experiences of homelessness, from the perspectives of Aboriginal and non-Aboriginal male and female service users in Adelaide, South Australia. In this chapter, I argue that an intersectional social work approach can make visible complex experiences of homelessness, by intersecting at least two categories of difference (Hulko, 2015). In documenting literature and research on the 'voices' and experiences of service users and people affected by homelessness, I explore the effects of colonisation and racism (particularly on Aboriginal Australians), debates about race relations, gendered aspects of homelessness, heterosexual dominance, age differences (such as older people, children and youth) and migration and refugee issues. I note that the perspectives of people who experience homelessness are often ignored (or re-constructed for particular political purposes), and advocate for more service user-led research.

The concluding chapter pulls together the strands of this book about the interrelationships between intersectionality, homelessness and social work. I make the claim that intersectionality can provide a new way of thinking about homelessness, social work research, social policy making and analysis, practitioner responses and service user perspectives. As such, an intersectional social work approach is a new way of moving forward towards inclusive approaches to homelessness, which incorporate diversity and listen to the voices of people most affected by homelessness.

Conclusion

There is already considerable multidisciplinary literature on homelessness and intersectionality. However, there is limited scholarship on intersectional and social work approaches to homelessness. In this chapter, I positioned this book within the complexities of intersectionality, homelessness and social work. I explained my argument and what intersectionality can offer to the fields of homelessness and social work. This chapter sets the context for the following chapters in the book that: further theorise intersectionality, discuss social work and intersectional research on homelessness, highlight multidisciplinary intersectional policy approaches, reflect on social work practice and make visible lived experiences and perspectives on homelessness.

Note

1 *Principles and Recommendations for Population and Housing Censuses*, Sales No. E.98.XVII.8 United Nations 1998 Paragraph 1.328.

References

Bacchi, C. (2009). *Analysing policy: What's the problem represented to be?* Frenchs Forest, NSW: Pearson.

Christensen, A. and Jensen, S. (2012). Doing intersectional analysis: Methodological implications for qualitative research. *Nordic Journal of Feminist and Gender Research*, 20(2), 109–125.

Crenshaw, K. (1991). Mapping the margins: Intersectionality, identity politics, and violence against women of color. *Stanford Law Review*, 43, 1241–1299.

Damant, D., Lapierre, S., Kouraga, A., Fortin, A., Hamelin-Brabant, L., Lavergne, C. and Lessard, G. (2008). Taking child abuse and mothering into account: Intersectional feminism as an alternative for the study of domestic violence. *Affilia: Journal of Women and Social Work*, 23, 123–133.

Dhamoon, R. (2011). Considerations on mainstreaming intersectionality. *Political Research Quarterly*, 64(1), 230–243.

Dominelli, L. (2002). Anti oppressive practices in context. (pp. 3–20). In R. Adams, L. Dominelli and M. Payne (Eds). *Social work themes, issues and critical debates* (2nd ed.). New York, NY: Palgrave Macmillan.

Dunk-West, P. (2013). *How to be a social worker: A critical guide for students.* Basingstoke, UK: Palgrave Macmillan.

Emslie, M. (2011). Youth housing workers and housing affordability: Living on Struggle Street. *Australian Social Work*, 64(3), 361–376.

Gibelman, M. (1999). The search for identity: Defining social work – Past, present, future. *Social Work*, 44(4), 298–310.

Gordon, L. and Zufferey, C. (2013). Working with diversity in a neoliberal environment. *Advances in Social Work and Welfare Education*, 15(1), 20–30.

Habitat. (2015). *World Habitat Day Key Housing Facts.* Accessed 21 April 2016. www.habitat.org/getinv/events/world-habitat-day/housing-facts.

Hankivsky, O. (Ed.). (2012). *An intersectionality-based policy analysis framework.* Vancouver, BC: Institute for Intersectionality Research and Policy, Simon Fraser University.

Hulko, W. (2009). The time-and context-contingent nature of intersectionality and interlocking oppressions. *Affilia: Journal of Women and Social Work*, 24(1), 44–55.

Hulko, W. (2015). Operationalizing intersectionality in feminist social work research: Reflections and techniques from research with equity seeking groups (pp. 69–90). In S. Wahab, B. Anderson-Nathe and C. Gringeri (Eds). *Feminisms in Social Work Research.* New York, NY: Routledge.

Lutz, H., Herrera Vivar, M.T., and Supik, L. (2011). *Framing intersectionality: Debates on a multi-faceted concept in gender studies.* Burlington, VT: Ashgate.

Lykke, N. (2010). *Feminist studies: A guide to intersectional theory, methodology, and writing.* New York, NY: Routledge.

McKay, T. and Zufferey, C. (2015). 'A who doing a what'? Identity, practice and social work education. *Journal of Social Work*, 15(6), 644–661.

McKibbin, G., Duncan, R., Hamilton, B., Humphreys, C. and Kellett, C. (2015).The intersectional turn in feminist theory: A response to Carbin and Edenheim (2013). *European Journal of Women's Studies*, 22(1), 99–103.

Masocha, S. (2015). *Asylum seekers, social work and racism.* Basingstoke, UK: Palgrave Macmillan.

May, V.M. (2015). *Pursuing intersectionality: unsettling dominant imaginaries.* New York, NY: Routledge.

Mehrotra, G. (2010). Toward a continuum of intersectionality theorizing for feminist social work scholarship. *Affilia: Journal of Women and Social Work*, 25(4), 417–430.

Murphy, Y., Hunt, V., Zajicek, A.M., Norris, A.N. and Hamilton, L. (2009). *Incorporating intersectionality in social work practice, research, policy, and education.* Washington, DC: National Association of Social Workers (NASW) Press.

Payne, M. (2014). *Modern social work theory* (4th ed.). New York, NY: Palgrave Macmillan.

Phoenix, A. and Pattynama, P. (2006). Editorial: Intersectionality. *European Journal of Women's Studies*, 13(3), 187–192.

Pulkingham, J., Fuller, S. and Kershaw, P. (2010). Lone motherhood, welfare reform and active citizen subjectivity. *Critical Social Policy*, 30(2), 267–291.

Shardlow, S. (2009). Values, ethics and social work. (pp. 37–46). In R. Adams, L. Dominelli and M. Payne (Eds). *Social work themes, issues and critical debates* (3rd ed.). New York, NY: Palgrave Macmillan.

Thornton Dill, B. and Kohlman, M.H. (2012). Intersectionality. (pp. 154–171). In S. Hesse-Biber (Ed.). *Handbook of feminist research*. Los Angeles, CA: Sage.

Thornton Dill, B. and Zambrana, R.E. (2009). *Emerging intersections: Race, class, and gender in theory, policy, and practice*. Piscataway, NJ: Rutgers University Press.

Tipple, G. and Speak, S. (2009). *The hidden millions: Homelessness in developing countries*. New York, NY: Routledge.

Tomas, A. and Dittmar, H. (1995). The experience of homeless women: An exploration of housing histories and the meaning of home. *Housing Studies*, 10(4), 493–513.

United Nations General Assembly. (1948). *Universal Declaration of Human Rights* (Article 25). Accessed 30 May 2013. www.ohchr.org/EN/UDHR/.

United Nations Human Rights Office of the High Commissioner. (2016). *Homelessness as a global human rights crisis that demands an urgent global response. Summary of the Report of the Special Rapporteur on the right to adequate housing, Leilani Farha*. Accessed 20 April 2016. www.ohchr.org/EN/Issues/Housing/Pages/AnnualReports.aspx.

Wahab, S., Anderson-Nathe, B. and Gringeri, C. (Eds) (2015). *Feminisms in social work research*. New York, NY: Routledge.

Wendt, S. and Moulding, N. (Eds) (2016). *Contemporary feminisms in social work practice*. Abingdon, UK: Routledge.

Winker, G. and Degele, N. (2011). Intersectionality as multi-level analysis: Dealing with social inequality. *European Journal of Women's Studies*, 18(1), 51–66.

Yuval-Davis, N. (2006). Intersectionality and feminist politics. *European Journal of Women's Studies*, 13(3), 193–209.

Yuval-Davis, N. (2012). Dialogical epistemology: An intersectional resistance to the 'Oppression Olympics'. *Gender and Society*, 26, 46–64.

Zufferey, C. (2007). *Homelessness, social work, social policy and the print media in Australian cities*, Phd Thesis. School of Social Work and Social Policy, University of South Australia.

Zufferey, C. (2008). Responses to homelessness in Australian cities: Social worker perspectives. *Australian Social Work*, 61(4), 357–371.

Zufferey, C. (2009). Making gender visible: Social work responses to homelessness. *Affilia: Journal of Women and Social Work*, 24(4), 382–393.

Zufferey, C. (2013). 'Not knowing that I do not know and not wanting to know': Reflections of a white Australian social worker. *International Social Work*, 56(5), 659–673.

Zufferey, C. (2015). Intersectional feminism and social work responses to homelessness. (pp. 90–103). In S. Wahab, B. Anderson-Nathe and C. Gringeri (Eds). *Feminisms in social work research*. New York, NY: Routledge.

Zufferey, C. (2016a) Homelessness and gender. In N. Naples, R. Hoogland, M. Wickramasinghe and A. Wong (Eds). *The Wiley-Blackwell encyclopedia of gender and sexuality studies*. DOI: 10.1002/9781118663219.wbegss010.

Zufferey, C. (2016b). Homelessness and intersectional feminist practice. (pp. 238–249). In S. Wendt and N. Moulding (Eds). *Contemporary feminisms in social work practice*. Abingdon, UK: Routledge.

Zufferey, C. and Chung, D. (2006). Representations of homelessness in the Australian print media: Some implications for social policy. *Just Policy*, 42, 33–38.

Zufferey, C. and Kerr, L. (2004). Identity and everyday experiences of homelessness: Some implications for social work. *Australian Social Work*, 57(4), 343–353.

2 Homelessness and social work

An intersectional approach

This chapter examines intersectionality in multidisciplinary literature, including social work, sociology, political science and women and gender studies. I present epistemological debates in intersectionality literature, along with critiques of the concept. I argue that diverse intersectional theorising can be integrated into social work approaches to homelessness to transcend individual and structural debates in homelessness and social work literature. Finally, I further discuss critiques, dilemmas and complexities of intersectionality, including McCall's (2005) categorical approaches, and Lykke's (2010) 'post-constructionist' theorising of intersectionality.

Background

American, Australian, British and European authors have tended to focus on homelessness by counting numbers of 'homeless people'; constructing objective policy definitions associated with particular resources; examining the causes of homelessness; calculating costs to the community; emphasising individual characteristics, needs and problems; finding solutions and highlighting transitions and pathways into and exiting from homelessness (Blau, 1992; Jencks, 1994; Johnson, 1995; Johnson and Cnaan, 1995; Clapham, 2002; 2005; Johnson *et al.*, 2008; Zufferey, 2008; Busch-Geertsema *et al.*, 2010). In this book I argue that intersectionality can challenge homogenous and linear representations of homelessness and complicate approaches that count numbers, construct objective definitions, examine singular causes, calculate costs, find solutions and highlight transitions and pathways. An intersectional approach can focus on power relations and how homelessness is multidimensional and inextricably connected to intersecting sites of disadvantage and inequality.

Social workers have also been criticised for homogenising and categorising people who are homeless and constructing causation discourses that do not fit the complexities of their lived experiences (Zufferey and Kerr, 2004; Horsell, 2006). Whilst focusing on individualised care issues and pathways into and out of homelessness can be useful responses, they do tend to emphasise how individual characteristics, needs and problems (such as substance abuse or mental illness) contribute to causing homelessness. This focus potentially supports individualist discourses and can obscure diverse and intersecting relations of power. Social workers, however, are involved in constructing both individualised and structural responses to homelessness, as well as building coalitions with service users in collaborative dialogues that work towards social justice (Zufferey, 2008; Mostowska, 2014). In this book, I argue that the individual-structural debates in homelessness and social work can be transcended by incorporating a multilayered conceptualisation of intersectionality (Winker and Degele, 2011).

Social work authors Murphy and her colleagues (2009) note that intersectionality provides a systems-focused perspective, which is consistent with social work's commitment to system reform and social justice. Thus, an intersectional social work approach helps frame social work advocacy efforts, through understanding how unequal power relations interplay to constitute social constructions of homelessness and social work responses to homelessness.

In this book I also contend that assumptions underpinning intersectionality are consistent with social work's commitment to social change and building coalitions between key stakeholders, such as researchers, policy makers, service providers and service users.

Intersectionality literature has variously focused on identity categories (or subjectivities) as well as meaning-making processes and how identities are socially located. This includes a focus on 'identities and categories of difference'; 'processes and systems of differentiation' and the 'complexities of subject formation' (Dhamoon, 2011, p. 231). These intersecting identity relations, social locations and structural barriers continue to constitute multiple forms of oppression (Crenshaw, 1991; Mehrotra, 2010), which contribute to shaping homelessness. This book posits that intersectionality enables social workers to recognise, examine, reflect on and address complex and multiple intersecting layers of 'oppression' (and privilege) that constitute social work and homelessness, including identity and process dynamics associated with gender, race, ethnicity, culture, class, sexuality, age and ability (Thornton Dill and Kohlman, 2012).

Intersectionality

Since the late nineteenth century, intersectional theorising has been promoted by black feminists, including Anna Julia Cooper's (1892) analysis of racism and sexism, Angela Davis' (1971) analysis of race, gender and class in black women's lives, Deborah King's (1988) discussion of multiple jeopardy and Patricia Hills Collins' (1990) theorising of the matrix of domination. Legal professor Kimberlie Crenshaw (1991) originally conceptualised structural and political intersectionality to respond to race and gender discrimination in the American legal context. This approach was initially established to understand how singular axes (such as gender or race) in anti-discrimination legislation ignored the multiple discriminations experienced by black women. The ways that gender intersects with other forms of inequality (especially those founded on racism and colonialism) has been under-theorised (Jackson and Scott, 2010), especially in social work. However, intersectional approaches go beyond gender and race locations, 'to any grouping of people, advantaged as well as disadvantaged' (Yuval-Davis, 2006, p. 201).

Intersectionality has been taken up by many different disciplines besides the legal profession (Crenshaw, 1991; 2003), including in women and feminist studies (Davis, 2008; Lykke, 2010; Carbin and Edenheim, 2013), political science (Wilson, 2013), by critical race theorists (King, 1988; hooks, 1990, 2000; Collins, 2000), as well as in social work (Murphy *et al.*, 2009). In the field of social work, intersectionality has tended to be used in a structuralist way, to forward a social justice agenda – such as to examine how social inequalities such as racism, sexism, classism, heterosexism, ableism and ageism are mutually constitutive and interact at micro (individual), mezzo (group) and macro (society) levels (Murphy *et al.*, 2009, p. 10). Intersectional approaches invite social workers to think simultaneously at the level of structures, dynamics and subjectivities (Carbin and Edenheim, 2013).

Intersectionality also 'emerged from feminist debates about difference at a particular historical moment in western culture' (McKibbin *et al.*, 2015, p. 101). Feminist approaches and social work have a long and intertwined history, sharing commitments to activism and the betterment of society (Kemp and Brandwein, 2010; Wahab *et al.*, 2015; Wendt and Moulding, 2016; Bryant, 2016). Feminist scholars encourage a reflexive positioning and a focus on situated knowledges, from diverse, multidisciplinary perspectives and locations (Lykke, 2010). Feminist movements have historically been constructed as 'waves'. For example, feminists of the second wave movement in the 1960s advocated for political and legal reform, and argued that women's oppression was related to unequal capitalist and patriarchal systems (Kemp and Brandwein, 2010). This movement included a commitment to women's emancipation and addressing oppressive and hierarchical power relations, such as sexism, homophobia, racism and religious oppression. These positions constitute what is known as critical or structural feminist approaches that have been criticised for constructing grand narratives and truths about oppression and binary power relations (Fawcett *et al.*, 2000). Furthermore, both feminism and social work have been criticised for promoting white, Western, middle-class women's experiences and neglecting to acknowledge diversity (hooks, 2000; Pease, 2010). Postcolonial and transnational feminist theorist Mohanty (2003), in her key text on ethnicity, argued that white, Western and middle-class feminists construct a homogenous global feminist 'we', with its origins in the privilege of whiteness.

Postmodern and post-structural feminism emerged from the criticism of critical and structural approaches. The postmodern feminist perspective is particularly associated with the work of Judith Butler (1990) who viewed gender as being discursively constructed and performative, while the term post-structural feminism focused more on discursive constructions of 'reality' and how language and discourses constitute gendered subjectivities within shifting power relations (Weedon, 1987). However, postmodern and post-structural feminisms have also been criticised for tending towards individualism, relativism and not providing a basis for collective political action (Fawcett *et al.*, 2000). From its inception, intersectional theorising was radical and political, it critiqued the essentialism of white identity-based politics, by highlighting the inseparability of racial and gender oppressions from the socio-political location and standpoint of black feminists (Mehrotra, 2010, p. 420; May, 2015).

Intersectional feminism has become a powerful discourse and useful political tool to disrupt dominant power relations (Yuval-Davis, 2006; Dhamoon, 2011; McKibbin *et al.*, 2015; May, 2015). Intersectional feminism incorporates numerous critiques of previous feminist approaches and is often now 'presented as *the* feminist theory' (Carbin and Edenheim, 2013, p. 245). Intersectionality is variously referred to as a framework (McCall, 2005; Hancock, 2007), a politics (Crenshaw, 1991), a metaphor (Crenshaw, 1991), a 'knowledge project' about a 'matrix of domination' (Collins, 2000), a theory (Yuval-Davis, 2006), a paradigm (Hancock, 2007), an analytical tool (Nash, 2008), a nodal point (Lykke, 2010), a discourse (McKibbin *et al.*, 2015) and a field (Carbin and Edenheim, 2013). Within the literature, authors note that there is a slippage in intersectionality theorising, between structuralist and poststructuralist ontologies, creating confusion about intersectional definitions (Carbin and Edenheim, 2013; McKibbin *et al.*, 2015).

Different countries and continents have engaged with intersectionality differently. In the American context, intersectionality has emerged from structuralist traditions, whilst in the British and European context, intersectional authors have tended to draw more on constructivist theorising (Carbin and Edenheim, 2013, p. 235). For three decades British sociologist Nira Yuval-Davis has published extensively on intersections between gender, ethnicity, race, class and nationality, and has advocated for broadening the 'triple oppression' (gender, race, class) argument of US-based black feminists. She argues for an intersectional approach that 'analyzes social stratification as a whole' and that we cannot homogenise the ways that any 'political project' affects different people (Yuval-Davis, 2011, p. 3). Recently, a group of Australian feminist (including some social workers) stated that they preferred to refer to intersectionality as being a 'discourse', to progress 'research, policy and practice responses to family violence and to other issues affecting disadvantaged groups of people' (McKibbin *et al.*, 2015, p. 102), which would include homelessness.

Dutch feminist and political philosopher Baukje Prins (2006) examines systemic (mostly US-based) and constructionist (mostly UK- and Europe-based) approaches to intersectionality. She notes that systemic intersectionality foregrounds structural inequalities, intersecting systems of domination/ subordination (related to, for example, gender, class, race, ethnicity and sexuality), and problematises binaries such as masculinity–femininity, white–black, middle–working class. However, constructionist authors argue that systemic approaches fall short in their analysis of agency and subjectivity and social identification constraints (Prins, 2006'; Lykke, 2010). That is, that constructionist approaches provide more possibilities for examining the complexities of intersectional identification, by taking into account both intersecting systems of power, and how power is subjectively productive and produced (Lykke, 2010). For example, how do intersecting power differentials produce individual life history narratives of both people who experience homelessness and social workers? How do social workers and people defined as homeless engage with these power dynamics? How are diverse experiences of homelessness affected by interwoven gendering, racialising, ethnifying and class stratifying processes? In this book, researchers, policy makers, social workers and activists are invited to consider their own social positions and power when taking an intersectional approach (see Chapter 5). I argue that multi-layered analyses that link individual experiences to broader structures and systems are crucial for exploring how power relations are shaped and experienced.

Intersectional scholars in social work literature advocate for including different analyses of neglected intersections. For example, similar to Yuval Davis, in a global context, Mehrotra (2010) maintains that intersectional social work must increasingly incorporate discussions on migration, diaspora and nationality. Sandberg (2013, p. 351) suggests that intersectional social work must also think about the meanings of local geographies and how this impacts on our analyses of and responses to social problems. Sandberg (2013, p. 351) argues that 'differences between urbanity and rurality are not only a matter of distribution of resources ... but are also linked to the privileges of definition that come with being situated as either at the centre or at the periphery'. For example, the omission of the voices of rural victims of domestic violence and rural social problems more widely reflects how rural issues are in a peripheral position, outside the centre of knowledge production in social work. Whilst urban and rural geographies cannot be conceptualised as an axis of oppression, rural locations can create particular kinds of vulnerability, such as isolation from services and supports (Sandberg, 2013), including in the field of homelessness (Cloke and Milbourne, 2006). Therefore, urban and rural geographies should be included when analysing neglected points of intersection and the diversity of people's lives (Sandberg, 2013). This applies to many neglected concepts in the field of social work and homelessness, including global and local migration, definitional differences and how intersecting experiences of sexuality, gender, ethnicity, race, age and class shape how homelessness and social work are constituted.

Multidisciplinary intersectionality scholars argue that 'social divisions have different organising logics' (Phoenix and Pattynama, 2006, p. 187) but that they are not independent and dichotomous. For example, socio-economic backgrounds, institutionalised racism, sexism and homophobia are ontologically different, with variable intersecting effects on the subjectivities of people who experience homelessness. British sociologists Strid *et al.* (2013, p. 575) argue that inequalities are interconnected but 'can simultaneously be named separately and distinguished', so that the relations between multiple inequalities are theorised as 'mutually shaping rather than as either additive or mutually constitutive'. Intersectional approaches explore social categories, social positions, social locations and normalising practices (Verloo, 2006), with the aim to construct a particular political project (May, 2015). The social construction of lived categories (such as gender, race/ethnicity, sexual orientation and class) are produced (and reproduced), in relation to a range of social positions (such as multiple ethnicities or dichotomised genders), the origins of the social category (such as the contested nature/nurture gender debates), the location of inequality (such as in regards to the organisation of labour, citizenship or intimacy), as well as the material and discursive processes that re-produce inequalities, in regards to white, heterosexual and middle-class norms (Verloo, 2006, p. 217). Intersectional authors call for a dialogue between people from different social positionings (Ferree, 2009; Yuval-Davis, 2012, p. 48). This would include social workers having a dialogue with people who are defined as 'homeless' about their experiences of homelessness, highlighting their perceptions of social workers and services (see Chapter 6).

An intersectional social work approach provides a new critical way of examining homelessness, by analysing and reflecting on intersecting power dynamics that are structural, political and cultural (Crenshaw, 1991). When Crenshaw spoke of the General Motors and African American women legal case that did not fit gender or race anti-discrimination laws, this has been referred to as an example of structural and political intersectionality (Lykke, 2010). She also discussed the numerous structural, political and representational interactions of race and gender in male violence against 'women of color' (Crenshaw, 1991). Next, I consider this framework in relation to social work and homelessness. First, structural inequalities are embodied, socio-political and experienced differently by different individuals. For example, homelessness is a structural issue caused by a myriad of interrelated injustices that social workers could work towards changing. However, each individual has different experiences of these inequalities, which requires different responses. Second, the political aspect of intersectionality can relate to how different categories of citizens engage in identity politics in ways that may disempower and marginalise each other unintentionally. For example, feminist advocates who focus entirely on gender can neglect how homelessness is constituted by a diverse range of interrelated social identities that have differing effects, dependent on the social and environmental contexts of individual lives. Lastly, cultural representations of homelessness can also disempower and reproduce gendered and racialised inequalities. For example, in my research on representations of homelessness in the Australia print media, it was evident that service providers were constructed as 'experts' and 'saints' who were 'helping' deserving people (Zufferey and Chung, 2006; Zufferey, 2012), which reinforced unequal power relations. Public discourses have tended to promote individualist explanations of homelessness and neglected to consider broader structural, political and social influences on how homelessness is represented and responded to (Horsell, 2006; Zufferey, 2008), which potentially shapes how the problem has come about and how social work responds to it.

Whilst Crenshaw is more structuralist in her approach, Lykke (2010, p. 51) draws on 'post -constructionist' ideas to define intersectionality as a theoretical and methodological tool for analysing unjust social relations. Lykke (2010) combines post-constructionist and corpomaterial (that is, the embodiment of sex and materiality of bodies) feminist approaches, including the semiotic-material approach of Haraway (1991) and discursive-material approach of Barad (2007). Her discussion of intersectionality weaves together ontology, epistemology and ethics, constructing ambiguity, multiplicity and diversity, as pluralist understandings (Lykke, 2010, p. 161). Lykke (2010) analyses how historically specific power relations (or 'constraining normativities') are based on discursive and structurally constricted social categories that interact to reproduce social inequalities. She argues that constructions of gender/biological sex intersect with other socioculturally constructed identities, such as race, ethnicity, class, sexuality, age, disability and nationality. In this book I explore both structuralist and poststructuralist conceptualisations of intersectionality, relating these to what they can offer to the theorising of social work and homelessness – because there has been considerable literature published on the topic of intersectionality, but not particularly in relation to social work and homelessness (Zufferey, 2009; Zufferey, 2015). I take both a critical and a social constructionist position to argue that intersectional theorising can provide a more robust approach from which to explore the diversities and complexities of homelessness, whilst also focusing on advocating for social justice and social change.

Social work and homelessness

The purpose of social work is related to 'helping' socially disadvantaged population groups and advocating for social change (AASW, 2010). Early social work authors constructed individual service needs of homeless persons as being basic, stabilisation needs, such as help in obtaining public entitlements and professional services; change-oriented needs, such as counselling and case management; and emergency needs, such as responding to crises (Johnson and Cnaan, 1995, p. 354). These individualised service responses and social work interventions have been aligned to policy and funding approaches that categorise the 'support needs' of 'homeless people', around housing, income, health, mental health, substance abuse and domestic and family violence. These approaches are also directed at population groups, such as men, women, children and families and/or focusing on geographical locations, such as rural and urban homelessness. However, these categorisation processes can contribute to 'siloing' or 'dichotomising' social work responses to homelessness, without focusing on how social inequalities are produced and intersect, to constitute social work responses to homelessness.

Whilst there are many social work scholars who have drawn on critical and structural approaches to homelessness, social work literature has historically been dominated by clinical approaches and medical discourses (Johnson and Cnaan, 1995). In the 1990s, American social work authors Johnson and Cnaan (1995, p. 340) provided an overview of social work involvement in the field of homelessness focusing on 'interventions' rather than sociological points of view. Johnson and Cnaan (1995, p. 341) synthesised articles published in social work literature, with at least one author who was a social worker, based on research that took place in social work settings, as well as widely cited 'classical studies' on homelessness. They found that most sources of information on homelessness focused on definitions, causes and cost to society – including moral cost – the composition of the homeless population, the needs of 'homeless people', treatment interventions and gaps in services (Johnson and Cnaan, 1995, p. 341; see also Hopper, 1989; Rossi, 1989; Blasi, 1990). This interventionist focus shapes contemporary social work responses to homelessness because discourses about 'individualised needs' are powerful in social work and homelessness literature (Zufferey, 2008; 2012). Focusing predominantly on gender, critical feminist Nancy Fraser (1989, p. 147) had argued that women are most likely to be service users and therefore, the 'needs' interpretation of the 'welfare client' is a feminised terrain that frequently positions them as passive recipients of social assistance. In this book, I argue that intersectionality can contribute to highlighting how *intersecting* social locations and social processes can both oppress and privilege service users and social workers, within unequal power relations.

Similarly, European social scientist Nordfeldt (2012, p. 117) promotes an intersectional approach to homelessness to capture complexity and consider intersections between structural, institutional and individual contexts that can increase the risk of people becoming homeless. These individual/structural debates have a long history in social work literature. Individualised discourses are frequently juxtaposed with structuralist explanations for homelessness (Horsell, 2006). British author Neale (1997) linked the concepts of undeserving and deserving to individual and structural discourses. She argued that when homelessness is interpreted as a function of structural factors, 'homeless people' are constructed as 'deserving' of services and assistance. However, individuals can equally be constructed as 'undeserving', if perceived to be responsible for their own homelessness. Taking this further, American sociologist Rosenthal (2000) observed that people who experience homelessness are labelled 'slackers' (incompetent because of their own fault, such as drugs users), 'lackers' (incompetent due to no fault of their own, such as people with a serious mental illness) and 'unwilling victims' (competent but caught in circumstance beyond their control, such as women escaping domestic violence). Rosenthal notes that to be 'deserving' of assistance requires one to be incompetent. This analysis points to disabling discourses in social work responses to homelessness. British social policy author Pleace (2000) argues that there is a 'new orthodoxy' in homelessness literature that combines structural/individual explanations of homelessness. That is, structural factors such as economic inequalities, poverty, unemployment and lack of affordable housing can create the conditions within which homelessness occurs – but some individuals are more vulnerable to the effects of these adverse social and economic conditions than others, which explains why more people with 'high support needs' experience homelessness (Pleace, 2000). Consistent with the approaches of sociologists Anthias (2001 and 2002) and Winker and Degele (2011), I posit that this debate can be taken further by proposing a multilayered intersectional social work approach that responds to: individual and group experiences of discrimination, social structures, interactions and processes, institutionalised organisational practices, cultural symbols and discursive representations of social problems, such as media representations of homelessness.

Intersectionality can also be used to understand and analyse political resistances that are intertwined with power relations that re-signify categories and normative identity markers (Lykke, 2010, p. 52). An intersectional social work approach advocates for social workers engaged in research, policy, practice and academia to reflect on what categories we privilege and what categories we make invisible. As well, how do individuals resist and negotiate the power relations and social conditions in which they are embedded? That is, how do people who are defined as homeless resist dominant definitions and public representations, often also promoted by social workers? These are perpetual reflexive questions for social workers working in the field of homelessness.

To represent intersectionality graphically, social work authors Murphy *et al.* (2009, p. 55) and Hulko (2015, p. 72) use circular diagrams illustrating intersections between multiple social locations and social identity categories, such as race, ethnicity, age, gender, class, physical ability, Indigeneity, nationality, sexuality, religion and so on. However, they position oppression and privilege in the circle differently. Murphy *et al.* (2009, pp. 54–55) place oppression at the centre of the circle and privilege on the outer edge, arguing that intersectional research often examines 'non-normative' population groups. This attention tends to align with feminists who focus on intersectional analysis as specific to black and ethnic minority women and 'marginalised' people/s (Murphy *et al.*, 2009).

Social work scholar Hulko (2015, p. 71) places privilege at the centre of the circle because she argues that intersectional research need not be restricted to people who inhabit multiple sites of oppression and marginalisation. When teaching about intersectionality, Hulko (2015) asks students to position themselves within a social location diagram. To define oppression, Hulko draws on Iris Marion Young's (2011) five faces of oppression: violence, exploitation, marginalisation, powerlessness and cultural imperialism. Hulko's approach is akin to the 'majority inclusive principle' of intersectionality (Christensen and

Jensen, 2012), which, I argue, enables social workers to reflect on their own privileges when working in the field of homelessness (see Chapter 5).

When discussing feminism and intersectional theory, Gina Samuels and Fariyal Ross-Sheriff (2008, p. 6) pose three challenges for scholars engaging in the intellectual agenda of intersectionality:

> [to] avoid essentialising the added groupings or identities of race, class, sexuality ... [to] attend to interlocking privileges as well as oppressions and ... [to] attend to changes in context that then shift the meaning of various social identities and statuses.

Ross Sheriff's work with Afghan women and Samuels' research with black-white racial adoptees highlight women's multiple and shifting identities and capabilities, in spite of their oppressive life conditions (Samuels and Ross-Sheriff, 2008, p. 6).

In this book I also advocate for an intersectional social work approach that explores the interplay between privileges and oppressions. Thus, I claim that it is important for social workers to ask critical questions such as: who defines who is oppressed or privileged? Can one person be variously oppressed or privileged in different contexts?

Multiple theorising

While intersectionality has dominated women's studies, it has been far less prevalent in the fields of social work and homelessness. The *European Journal of Women's Studies* published a special issue on intersectionality after considerable debate on what constitutes intersectionality at their tenth anniversary conference (Phoenix and Pattynama, 2006). Given that there is not one feminist epistemology, the recognition of particular intersections has created much debate and tensions among multidisciplinary feminist scholars (Lykke, 2010). Despite diverse structural, systemic, constructionist, positional and discursive theorising within intersectional literature, mobilising and combining anti-racist, anti-sexist, anti-homophobic, anti-nationalist and anti-colonial movements remains important (Yuval-Davis, 2006; Bredstrom, 2006; Lykke, 2010; May, 2015). Next, I explore the diverse perspectives and research of multidisciplinary intersectional authors, namely Lykke (2010), Dhamoon (2011), Matsuda (1991), McCall's (2005) categorical approaches, Winker and Degele (2011) and May (2015).

Lykke's (2010, p. 87) work on intersectionality, in the context of the discipline of women and gender studies, takes a 'post-constructionist' approach to intersectionality. She notes that gender and other social categorisations are historically, socially, culturally and linguistically constructed. Lykke (2010, p. 68) provides a genealogical analysis of the concept of intersectionality. This genealogy shows that intersectionality was explicitly named by Crenshaw (1991). However, Lykke (2010) argues that even before this term was coined, the implicit focus on intersectionality, intersecting power differentials and normative identity markers, can be traced back to the nineteenth century. For example, Sojourner Truth's speech in 1851, 'Ain't I a woman?', foreshadows campaigns by black feminists more than a century later. As well, in 1977, the Combahee River Collective promoted a 'Black Feminist Statement' outlining the intersections between black women's political, sexual and economic oppressions (Kemp and Brandwein, 2010). Lykke (2010) argues that it is important to read history with intersectionality as a lens, even when the label or name was not used. That is, that feminist theorising of intersectionality has occurred under other names, using other concepts and frames.

Furthermore, feminist activism has provided a strong challenge to the legitimising of biologically determinist and culturally essentialist perceptions of sex/gender and other sociocultural categorisations (Lykke, 2010, p. 25). Stressing the importance of gender de-constructionist theories to challenge biological determinism and cultural essentialism, she argues that the constructionist agenda has been able to establish sociocultural gender as a specific area of knowledge independent of biological sex. Feminist deconstruction goes back to authors such as Simone De Beauvoir who argued that 'One is not born but becomes a woman' (1984 [1949]) and to Judith Butler (1990; 2004) who wrote about 'doing gender', linking queer, post-structuralism, deconstruction and speech act theory. Lykke (2010) discusses intersectional feminism from both postcolonial/anti-racist and queer feminist prongs, which challenges the exclusiveness of gendered and racialised power relations, but neglects to consider intersections, such as between ethnicity and hetero/sexuality. In this book I argue that unequal power relations are social processes in which gender intersects with other social locations (such as ethnicity and sexuality), with associated discourses and 'real' material effects. For example, men and women are socially located within different gendered and racialised power relations that intersect and contribute to maintaining homelessness (Passaro, 2014).

Political scientist Rita Dhamoon (2011, pp. 230–240) identifies changing considerations in intersectional literature. She argues that the spirit of critical self-reflection, concepts and language used in intersectional literature are subject to change. Various terms are used that describe intersections, including interlocking, multiple jeopardy, discrimination-within-discrimination, multiple consciousness (King, 1988; Matsuda, 1992), multiplicity (Wing, 1990–1991), multiplex epistemologies (Phoenix and Pattynama, 2006, p. 187), translocational positionality (Anthias, 2002), multidimensionality (Hutchinson, 2001), inter-connectivities (Valdes, 1995) and synthesis (Ehrenreich, 2002). Nonetheless, keeping the focus on interactions assists to examine how 'processes of differentiation *dynamically* function through one another ... although the character of these processes and their effects are varied and indeterminate' (Dhamoon, 2011, p. 231). For example, in social work, the process of differentiating who is and who is not homeless is contested and differs in different cultural contexts. Dhamoon (2011, p. 235) proposes that a swirling matrix of meaning making can pictorially capture the 'interactive, unbounded, and relational dynamics of productive power'. She argues that although difference making is 'shifting, messy, indeterminate, dynamic and multilayered', it does not preclude 'locating contingent specificities of difference and power' (Dhamoon, 2011, p. 239). I also propose that dynamic meaning-making processes are important for examining the complexities and diversities of social work and homelessness. However, social work decisions are made within specific social and geographical locations that intersect with normative gendered, racialised, sexualised, classed and able-bodied assumptions.

In legal studies, Matsuda (1991, p. 1189) argues that intersectionality assists us to examine the blind spots of an analysis. For example, when we see something that looks racist, we might ask, where is the patriarchy in this? Or, if something looks homophobic, ask, where is class? Such questions enable social workers to let implicit social relations frame questions of explicit intersectional analysis, to include missing or invisible categories. However, this process does not answer whether there is a finite or infinite list of intersections or whether categorisations may reinforce or neutralise each other. To the question of 'how many facets of social difference and axes of power need to be analysed?' Yuval-Davis' (2012, p. 3) answer is that the number depends upon time and place, and involves assessing empirical reality as well as political and ontological struggles. For the purposes of this book, an intersectional analysis of homelessness and social work will highlight the material and discursive diversities and complexities of the issue at this point in time.

Sociologist Leslie McCall (2005; 2009) is motivated by questions about how different kinds of explicit intersectional analysis handle the complexities of power differentials, as evident in her discussion of anti-categorical, intra-categorical and inter-categorical methodologies. I have previously examined these categorical complexities in relation to homelessness when discussing feminist social work research and practice (see Zufferey, 2015; 2016).

An anti-categorical approach examines how concepts, terms and categories are constructed, and problematises the processes of categorisation (McCall, 2005).This approach can deconstruct problematic categorisations and the fixing of homeless and social work identities, around for example, gender roles, racial differences, class disadvantage, age stereotypes and sexuality, which invites a rethinking and reconceptualising of social work and homelessness. For example, in Chapter 4, I deconstruct policy definitions of homelessness that highlight housing as a solution to homelessness. Dominant definitions can be deconstructed from the perspectives of women and children affected by domestic violence who experience feelings of homelessness in their own homes, as well as from the perspectives of Aboriginal people for whom Indigenous notions of 'home' are often unrelated to housing (Zufferey and Chung, 2015). This analysis can be done without essentialising and homogenising these differences as for example, male or female and Indigenous or non-Indigenous traits or 'characteristics', but by noting that homelessness is discursively constructed, with material effects. As well, in regards to geo-graphical location, Sandberg's (2013, p. 360) research on rural women's experiences of domestic violence found that anti-categorical approaches can deconstruct 'rural and urban as categories' as well as locate 'local geographies within discourses of power and knowledge'.

When discussing urban and rural geographical locations and intimate partner violence (IPV), Sandberg (2013) argues for combining intra- and anti-categorical approaches. This is so that rural victims of IPV are analysed as a neglected point of intersection and that the diversity of 'ruralities' are also acknowledged. She contends that the 'uncritical use of the category 'rural' in studies of IPV may contribute to the othering of rurality where negative stereotypes of being 'backward, dumb and violent hillbillies' are reproduced (Sandberg, 2013, p. 357). However, 'shifting between intra- and anti-categorical approaches requires a great deal of epistemological flex-ibility' (Sandberg, 2013, p. 360). This analysis by Sandberg indicates how McCall's (2005) different categorical approaches in intersectionality do not need to stand alone and can be combined, whilst continuing to align with social work's commitment to social justice and equality.

The intra-categorical focus takes the construction of identity categories (or social locations) into account but acknowledges that identities are fluid and multiple, and that intersections within social categories are neglected in research literature (McCall, 2005; Winker and Degele, 2011). The intra-categorical intersectional approach assists social workers to focus on neglected and diverse perspectives of different stakeholders in the field of homelessness in more depth. For example, by asking the questions: how are intersections associated with sexuality neglected (Rowntree, 2014) in social work literature and research on homelessness, when are they made visible, and from whose perspective?

Inter-categorical approaches tend to examine relationships of inequality between population groups and categories strategically, to explore 'the nature of the relationships of social groups and, importantly, how they are chang-ing' (McCall, 2009, p. 59). For example, regional and economic inequalities central to homelessness can be highlighted by examining different dimensions of wage inequalities in different regions of the United States (McCall, 2009). In this book I argue that each of these intersectional approaches can be use-ful for examining the complex power dynamics in social workers' responses to homelessness.

Nonetheless, intersectional theorists (such as social workers) are cau-tioned against constructing 'hierarchies of oppression' that centre 'single axis logics' (Yuval-Davis, 2012, p. 48; May, 2015, p. 63). Given that the purpose of social work has historically been related to empowerment and addressing injustice affecting socially disadvantaged groups (BASW, 2002; IFSW, 2005; NASW, 2008; AASW, 2010), when analysing 'difference' it is difficult for social workers to resist constructing additive, compounding ideas of disadvantage. If social workers engage in arguing about which social category is more or less oppressed, social workers are constructing hierarchies of disadvantage and competing in a process that Yuval Davis (2012, p. 48) calls the 'oppression olympics'. For example, if social workers are examining race and gender relations that contribute to homelessness, the homeless experiences of men, women and children from ethnic minority and Aboriginal population groups can be made visible, including their risks of remaining poor and becoming homeless. However, a missing question could be: where is dis/ability, religion, class, age and sexuality in this analysis (Matsuda, 1991)? Yet, it is also important not to homogenise people from, for example, ethnic minority groups or Aboriginal backgrounds, by also focusing on the diversities within population groups. Thus, the 'doing' of intersectional research, policy and practice is complicated, which can be further understood by engaging with McCall's (2005) anti-categorical, intra-categorical and inter-categorical approaches.

European sociologists Winker and Degele (2011) argue for a multi-layered intersectional analysis that incorporates and broadens McCall's (2005) categories. They contend that to engage in intersectionality involves thinking simultaneously at the level of structures, dynamics and subjectivities. They used intersectionality when analysing 13 narrative interviews with people with no paid employment, who were 'differentiated in terms of age, social origin, gender, sexual orientation, child responsibility, nationality, ethnicity, work experience, physical capability and so on' (Winker and Degele, 2011, p. 58). The eight steps of their intersectional analysis sought to: describe identity constructions (such as woman-man, poor-rich), identify symbolic representations (such as women are better communicators than men), find references to social structures (such as according to gender, class, race and the body), interrelate central categories (such as classism, sexism, racism, heteronormativism, bodyisms etc.), compare and cluster subject constructions (such as, control over one's bodily self, overcoming bureaucratic barriers, desiring a stake in society and financial security), analyse power dynamics, deepen analysis of injustice and elaborate on intersections, such as how constructions support or resist dominant norms (Winker and Degele, 2011, p. 63). These multilayered analytical processes are also particularly pertinent to social work and homelessness, to intersect individual, structural, political and representational explanations of homelessness, whilst advocating for social justice.

American women's studies scholar Vivian May (2015, p. x) focuses on social justice and social change and explains that intersectionality is:

> resistant knowledge developed to unsettle conventional mindsets, challenge oppressive power, think through the full architecture of structural inequalities and asymmetrical life opportunities, and seek a more just world. It has been forged in the context of struggles for social justice as a means to challenge dominance, foster critical imaginaries and craft collective models for change.

This explanation reinforces that it is crucial to frame intersectionality as a form of 'social critique to foreground its radical capacity to disrupt oppressive vehicles of power' (Dhamoon, 2011, p. 230). However, there are debates in literature about categorisation processes.

Categories and processes

Social work scholars such as Murphy *et al.* (2009) note that inclusive social work practice would be well served to incorporate McCall's (2005) categorical approaches. However, scholars such as Lykke (2010), influenced by post-isms (such as post-structuralism and post-constructionism), have argued that McCall's categorical classifications are limiting, especially when considering the nuances of intersectional inequalities. This more post-structural perspective aims to move beyond 'categorisations' to emphasise the power relations and social 'processes' contributing to social inequalities. That is, intersectionality involves categorisations that occur through constitutive processes that are gender*ing*, racialis*ing*, class*ing*, dis/able*ing* and 'third world*ing*' and which can be both oppressing and privileging (Bacchi, forthcoming). As McKibbin *et al.* (2015, p. 99) and Carbin and Edenheim (2013) remind us, intersectionality emerged from a structuralist ontology. However, McKibbin *et al.* (2015, p. 101) advocate for an intersectional feminism that draws on poststructuralist ontologies that can 'still hold a notion of subjectivity to be the experience of self as an effect of power and discourse'.

In intersectional theorising, there has been a shift from studying identities and categories to studying processes and systems, moving away from potentially essentialising identities and towards using the post-structural notion of subjectivities. Therefore, intersectionality can combine a focus on identities, categories, processes and systems to include:

> identities of an individual or set of individuals or social group that are marked as different (e.g., a Muslim woman or black women), the categories of difference (e.g., race and gender), the processes of differentiation (e.g., racialisation and gendering), and the systems of domination (e.g., racism, colonialism, sexism, and patriarchy).
>
> (Dhamoon, 2011, p. 240)

I would also argue that these intersecting identities, categories, processes and systems are important to consider in the fields of social work and homelessness. The process of marking and claiming identity differences involves examining how the identities of both 'homeless people' and 'social workers' are diversely constituted and embodied. Subjectivities are constituted by messy and intersecting power differentials, within social processes that can be both privileging and oppressing.

However, social work responses to homelessness exist within unequal power relations that potentially uphold the status quo. That is, social work practice exists within 'systems of domination' that are racist, colonialist, sexist and patriarchal, to name just a few (Dhamoon, 2011, p. 240). Therefore, it remains important for an intersectional social work approach to involve self-reflexivity, during which social workers reflect on their own privileged social location/s, in relation to people who experience homelessness. In social work practice, power is produced, relational and located within social institutions that function to include and exclude people through the construction of difference/s, such as social workers constructing who is deemed 'deserving' or 'undeserving' of services. In New York, Passaro (1996; 2014) examined how gender, race and family status contributed to chances of exiting homelessness. She found that remaining homeless is a different process to becoming 'houseless' and that black men were most likely to be chronically homeless because they were overlooked by the service system, pointing to gendered and racialised practices of social discrimination.

In contrast to this critical approach, drawing on post-structural theorising, Lykke (2010, p. 150) argues that intersectional theorising actually constructs provisional boundaries and defines how subjects and objects relate to each other, which differs according to each particular political project. She creates a dynamic world of research subjects, objects of knowledge, knowers and what is known, building on Haraway's (1991; 2004) and Barad's (1996) theorising. For example, Lykke (2010, p. 53) draws on Karen Barad's (2003, p. 815) notion of 'intra-action' to argue that identity categories are not bounded phenomena but processes of mutual construction and transformation, through interpersonal communication. Both the research subject and the object of research are defined and contextualised within the relationship between the two, not fixed but momentary (Lykke, 2010, p. 151). Lykke's (2010) work is also relevant to social work research and practice because constructions of intersubjectivities in interpersonal communication is an important process to consider for social workers working in the field of homelessness.

Furthermore, social work is a self-reflexive project. Haraway's notion of situated knowledges (1988) explores the interconnectedness between the *siting* and the *sighting* of research concepts (Lykke, 2010, p. 152), such as homelessness. The notion of *siting* involves the researcher reflecting on his/her situatedness in time, space, history, body and inscribed intersecting power differentials (Lykke, 2010). For example, unequal power relations position (or site) the social work researcher in the research process and contribute to how research topics are sighted. Nonetheless, research participants (such as people who are defined as homeless) are social agents whose actions are beyond the control of the researcher. As well, the interconnectedness of materials and discursive dimensions of research designs should be scrutinised because discourses and materiality are inseparable (Lykke, 2010, p. 152). According to Barad (1996), research is constructed as a result of the processes of 'siting' and 'sighting' (all influenced by the social worker's lens). These procedures can be seen to be a form of *situated intersectionality* (Yuval-Davis, 2015), whereby social processes and social locations can be privileging and/or oppressing, depending on the context, time and place of the interaction. These social processes can contribute to upholding or resisting dominant understandings of a particular social phenomenon, such as homelessness.

In contrast to producing reductionist distinctions between different categories, Lykke (2010, p. 153) draws on Haraway's (2004) metaphor of *implosion* to accentuate complexity, relationality, inseparability and interconnectedness. Implosion is a process that collapses inwards rather than outwards and can be traced back to dynamic processes of transformation, from which there are momentary products that are at the same time subjective and objective, discursive and material, organic and technological, as well as human and nonhuman (Lykke, 2010, p. 154). The world is a complex process and it is analytically problematic to sort out subjectivity from objectivity, discourses from materiality, fact from fiction and micro from macro (Lykke, 2010, p. 154). Building on notions of reflection and representation, the metaphor of *diffraction* is used by Haraway (1997) to disrupt linear, causal explanations of difference and to examine dynamic and complex social processes. This intersectional theorising of differencing processes through implosion and diffraction can potentially disrupt linear constructions of homelessness that assume a continuum, and one way progressions related to entry into and exiting from homelessness, to encompass more entangled and fluid constructions.

Therefore, whilst a reflexive methodology is like using a mirror as a critical tool, Lykke (2010, p. 154) argues that this does not bring us further than the 'static logic of the Same'. That is, we are not limited to reflecting on oneself (a 'social worker') in relation to 'the Other' (a 'homeless person'). Drawing on the works of Haraway (1997) and Barad (1996), as discussed previously, Lykke (2010) proposes that the notions of diffraction, together with imploded objects and siting and sighting phenomena, can examine the complex production of difference patterns and create new understandings of an ever-changing world. For example, when a research object (such as homelessness) can be interpreted as an imploding, diffracting object or phenomenon, the analysis can be diverse and multifaceted.

Lastly, Lykke (2010, p. 161) discusses how *ethics* differ according to feminist positions. The anti-epistemological approaches of postmodern feminisms are deconstructive and problematise categories, such as 'woman', 'experience' and 'standpoint', which cannot simply be defined as 'good' and 'just' (Lykke, 2010). Therefore, feminist (and social work) ethics do not involve framing the correct response to the socially constructed 'other' but rather involve responsibility and accountability for the 'lively relationalities of becoming' of which we are all part (Barad, 2007, pp. 377–393). These ideas are important for social workers researching homelessness, to move beyond commonly constructed us–them dichotomies that represent social workers and service users. Both homelessness and social work are temporally and spatially located, socially constructed concepts as well as material experiences, with diverse and intersecting social effects and consequences.

Lykke's (2010) intersectional theorising goes beyond McCall's (2005) categorisations, using a more post-constructionist and post-structural lens. However, both of these theorists can be useful for exploring and constructing intersectional social work approaches to homelessness. This book aims to incorporate intersectionality into social work and homelessness scholarship, rather than take a position on these debates in literature about intersectionality. Nonetheless, a brief discussion of the critiques of intersectionality is in order, given that they are flourishing (May, 2015) and engender the 'same disciplining moves among feminists that have been deployed against feminism' (Crenshaw, 2011, p. 223), especially against black feminists in the academy.

Critiques of intersectionality

Critiques of intersectionality involve questioning its 'theoretical, political and methodological adequacy' (May, 2015, p. 103). These include: that intersectional theorists continue to promote universal structural inequalities based on single axis approaches that centre on, for example, gender, race or social class; that it increases fragmentation; that it is not being 'rigorous' and systematic, and is becoming meaningless as a term (May, 2015, p. 105). That is, that intersectionality has become a 'catch-all phrase' (Phoenix and Pattynama, 2006, p. 187), and is not performing what it declares (Carbin and Edenheim, 2013, p. 240). Nash (2008, p. 4) notes that feminist and anti-racist scholars drawing on intersectionality must attend to 'difference while also strategically mobilizing the language of commonality'; that there is a ' lack of a defined intersectional methodology'; that 'black women are often used as quintessential intersectional subjects'; that intersectionality is vaguely defined, and that there are tensions in the 'empirical validity of intersectionality' (for example, is it a 'theory of marginalized subjectivity or a generalized theory of identity'?). Nonetheless, Nash (2008, p. 13) argues that 'privilege and oppression can be co-constituted' subjectively, and that Crenshaw's concept of intersectionality 'has galvanized an array of disciplines to consider questions of essentialism, exclusion, and complex identity in new ways'. Yet, Crenshaw's structural approach has also been critiqued by Lykke (2010) for being too static. Lykke (2010) argues that when an analysis of the subtle processes involved in discursively constructing multiple identity markers is necessary, Crenshaw's (2003) notion of crossroads is not sufficient, as it would be for legal advocacy work. She implicitly critiques scholars who assume an ethic of neutrality, as well as those who advocate from a standpoint, including the advocacy of black feminist standpoint theorists, such as Patricia Hill Collins (2000).

In turn, Lykke (2010) has been critiqued for focusing too strongly on gender and not enough on intersections, and for ignoring historical political struggles in feminism by marginalised groups (May, 2015). Her genealogical analysis, in which she shows that 'intersectional thinking' predates the concept of 'intersectionality', has been criticised for failing to:

incorporate the serious criticism from marginalized feminist groups from all over the world (black, lesbian, colonized) in the 1970s and 1980s ... reduced by only being acknowledged as examples of 'intersectional thinking' alongside white and heterosexual feminist 'intersectional thinking'.

(Carbin and Edenheim, 2013, p. 4)

Thus, Lykke's (2010) theorising of intersectionality has been criticised for lacking in specificity and content, and for failing to acknowledge the ongoing political struggles of minority women for social justice (Carbin and Edenheim, 2013).

As well, European feminist authors Carbin and Edenheim (2013, p. 245) position constructivist intersectionality within a particular neoliberal, sociopolitical context:

Intersectional feminism, and maybe especially its constructivist version, we fear, has come to signal a liberal consensus-based project (that ignores capitalism as oppressive structure) in an increasingly neoliberal and conservative European context.

As previously discussed, this positioning has been resisted by a group of Australian feminist authors, who note that intersectionality can be used collectively, even as a 'discourse' (McKibbin *et al.*, 2015, p. 101).

Some post-structural authors argue that Crenshaw's (1991) original intention in developing the term intersectionality, which was about how to map 'intersectional dynamics', is recaptured by post-structural feminists, who advocate for more complex metaphors (Bacchi and Eveline, 2010). As Crenshaw (1991, pp. 1296–1297) observes, 'to say that a category such as race or gender is socially constructed is not to say that that category has no significance in the world'. As well, 'power clusters around certain categories and is exercised against others', such that the claiming of an identity is one 'differencing practice' that may at times be necessary (Crenshaw, 1991, p. 1297; Bacchi and Eveline, 2010). However, I do not support the concept of intersectionality as being a static list of structural, social locations, as this can lead to essentialist, problematic identity politics. As Crenshaw (1991, p. 1242) maintains, identity politics can also conflate or ignore intragroup difference as markers of social inequality. Feminist post-structural scholars such as Lykke (2010) and Bacchi (2009) contend that there are multiple truths and realities, and that gendering, racialising, heteronorming and disabling social dynamics discursively interact. They emphasise the importance of challenging the essentialising of identities, whilst at the same time supporting collective action in the formation of identity groups, in response to harmful 'differencing' dynamics (Bacchi and Eveline, 2010). In relation to social work, an intersectional approach would mean that social workers reflect on their own privileges within these 'differencing' dynamics.

Danish social psychologist Dorthe Staunaes (2003) contends that the concept of intersectionality needs re-working to incorporate the agency of the subject. Although individuals (including social workers) are constrained by discourses, within these limits they also engage in meaning-making processes, take up subject positions, elaborate on them and make them their own. An intersectional analytical process can examine where different categorisations are taken up and prioritised in the everyday life experience of subjects, including social workers and people who experience homelessness. Different discursive normativities construct different constraints for differently gendered, ethnicised and racialised individuals, rather than 'predefined' grids of intersecting categories (Lykke, 2010, p. 74). Therefore, I contend that social workers would benefit by looking at processes by which individuals create meaning out of categorisations and normativities that frame everyday lives, rather than what people 'are' or 'have'. This involves examining the 'doing' of intersectionality and how this 'doing' results in troubled/untroubled (Wetherell, 1998) or inappropriate/d (Minh-ha, 1986) subject positions.

To conclude, according to sociologist Kathy Davis (2008), intersectionality is a meeting place for both structuralists and post-structuralists. Taking a different view, Bacchi (2012) maintains that melding different positions is a way of depoliticising social processes to make 'everyone' feel at home but in the end, some positions are prioritised and others are silenced. Bacchi (2012) notes that we cannot leave our ontological positions 'outside', which she believes is an ontological misunderstanding because how one sees the world clearly has consequences. She argues that conventional research projects displace ontological assumptions from the research process, 'even as they are implicitly central to them' (Bacchi in Bletsas and Beasley, 2012, p, 131). In this book, I invite readers to take up their own positions, by acknowledging that it depends on their political project, whether they incorporate structural or post-structural thought in their intersectional theorising. Like Ferree (2009), I am not arguing that *only* an intersectional analysis can do justice to the complexities of political power and social inequality. However, an intersectional social work approach can highlight that social inequalities intersect, are dynamic and are in changing, mutually constituted *relationships* with each other, from which they cannot be disentangled (Walby, 2007).

Conclusion

In this chapter, I have raised a number of questions about the applicability of intersectionality to social work and homelessness. The complexities of intersectionality and diverse scholarly engagement with the approach can be overwhelming and difficult to integrate. Intersectional theorising examines categorical complexities, multiple and intersecting axes of social difference and social processes that contribute to maintaining privilege and oppression (McCall, 2005; Yuval-Davis, 2006; Bryant and Hoon, 2006; Gressgård, 2008; Winker and Degele, 2011; Christensen and Jensen, 2012). However, I did ask myself, can this theorising be done without taking a position on whether there is a finite or infinite list of intersections, or on whether categorisations may reinforce or neutralise each other? Drawing on Lykke's (2010) use of Karen Barad's (2003, p. 815) notion of 'intra-action', I came to understand that identity is not a category or a bounded phenomenon, but is mutually constructed through social processes, that can be unjust or mutually transformative. This mutually transformative understanding can potentially occur through processes of interpersonal communication central to the skills, ethics and values of social work.

I have examined multidisciplinary intersectional literature and have argued for integrating an intersectional approach in social work responses to homelessness. The complexities of intersectionality make it a useful frame with which to view social work and homelessness. That is because diverse physical, emotional, spatial, ontological and spiritual contexts constitute experiences of homelessness (Somerville, 1992; 2013), as well as social work. Consistent with social justice ethics and anti-oppressive social work approaches, intersectional theorising involves locating and position-ing social work and homelessness within social institutions that are une-qual, multilayered, dynamic and complex (Mattsson, 2014). It can broaden activism in this area by challenging dichotomous powerless/powerful iden-tities constructed in client-worker relationships that frame homelessness as a social problem to be 'fixed' by service providers, such as social work-ers (Zufferey, 2008; Winker and Degele, 2011). Thus, intersectional social work approaches can be potentially transformative, by examining social processes, as well as intersecting social categorisations that can constitute social inequalities (Yuval-Davis, 2006, p. 201; Nixon and Humphreys, 2010, p. 138), such as homelessness.

A key consideration for social work practitioners, policy makers and educators in the fields of homelessness is to be well informed about the intersectional inequalities and discrimination affecting their client group/s. Yuval-Davis (2012, p. 48) calls for transformative dialogue between people from different positionings, which, in this context, includes social work prac-titioners, diverse groups of service users and policy makers. The challenge for social workers is to maintain a focus on how social processes and categorisa-tions intersect, to contribute to the constitution of the 'problem' of homeless-ness and how social work responds to it. This book is the first step towards examining intersectionality in social work and homelessness research, policy and practice, and towards advancing an intersectional social work approach to homelessness that is inclusive and respectful of diversity.

References

Anthias, F. (2001). The material and the symbolic in theorizing social stratification: Issues of gender, ethnicity and class. *British Journal of Sociology*, 52(3), 367–390.

Anthias, F. (2002). Beyond feminism and multiculturalism: Locating difference and the politics of location. *Women's Studies International Forum*, 25, 275–286.

Australian Association of Social Workers (AASW). (2010). *Code of ethics*. Accessed 10 March 2012. www.aasw.asn.au/document/item/740.

Bacchi, C. (2009). *Analysing policy: What's the problem represented to be?* Sydney: Pearson.

Bacchi, C. (2012). Introducing the 'What's the problem represented to be?' approach. (pp. 21–24). In A. Bletsas and C. Beasley (Eds). *Engaging with Carol Bacchi: Strategic interventions and exchanges*. Adelaide, SA: University of Adelaide Press.

Bacchi, C. (forthcoming). Policies as gendering practices: Re-viewing categorical distinctions. *Journal of Women, Politics and Policy*.

Bacchi, C. and Eveline, J. (2010). *Mainstreaming politics: Gendering practices and feminist theory*. Adelaide, SA: The University of Adelaide Press.

Barad, K. (1996). Meeting the universe halfway: Realism and social constructivism without contradiction. (pp. 161–194). In L.H. Nelson and J. Nelson *(Eds)*. *Feminism, science, and the philosophy of science*. Dordrecht; Boston, MA: Kluwer Academic Publishers.

Barad, K. (2003). Posthuman performativity: Towards an understanding of how matter comes to matter. *Signs: Journal of Women in Culture and Society*, 28(3), 801–831.

Barad, K. (2007). *Meeting the universe halfway: Quantum physics and the entanglement of matter and meaning*. Durham, NC: Duke University Press.

Blasi, G.L. (1990). Social policy and social science research on homelessness. *Journal of Social Issues*, 46, 207–219.

Blau, J. (1992). *The visible poor*. New York, NY: Oxford University Press.

Bletsas, A. and Beasley, C. (2012) *Engaging with Carol Bacchi. Strategic interventions and exchanges*. Adelaide, SA: University of Adelaide Press.

Bredstrom, A. (2006). Intersectionality: A challenge for feminist HIV/AIDS research? *European Journal of Women's Studies*, 13, 245–258.

British Association of Social Workers (BASW). (2002). *The code of ethics for social work*. Accessed 12 March 2012. http://cdn.basw.co.uk/membership/coe.pdf.

Bryant, L. (2016). Repositioning social work research in feminist epistemology, research and praxis. (pp. 82–98). In S. Wendt, and N. Moulding (Eds). *Contemporary feminisms in social work practice*. Abingdon, UK: Routledge.

Bryant, L. and Hoon, E. (2006). How can the intersections between gender, class, and sexuality be translated to an empirical agenda? *International Journal of Qualitative Methods*, 5(1), 6–11.

Busch-Geertsema, V., Edgar, W., O'Sullivan, E. and Pleace, N. (2010). Homelessness and homeless policies in Europe: Lessons from research. FEANTSA, European Consensus Conference on Homelessness, 9–10 December 2010, Brussels.

Butler, J. (1990). *Gender trouble: Feminism and the subversion of identity*. London: Routledge.

Butler, J. (2004). *Undoing gender*. New York, NY: Routledge.

Carbin, M. and Edenheim, S. (2013). The intersectional turn in feminist theory: A dream of a common language? *European Journal of Women's Studies*, 20, 233–248.

Christensen, A. and Jensen, S. (2012). Doing intersectional analysis: Methodological implications for qualitative research. *Nordic Journal of Feminist and Gender Research*, 20(2), 109–125.

Clapham, D. (2002). Housing pathways: A post modern analytical framework. *Theory and Society*, 19(2), 57–68.

Clapham, D. (2005). *The meaning of housing*. Bristol, UK: Policy Press.

Cloke, P. and Milbourne, P. (Eds) (2006). *International perspectives on rural homelessness*. New York, NY: Routledge.

Collins, P.H. (2000 [1990]). *Black feminist thought: Knowledge, consciousness, and the politics of empowerment* (2nd ed.). London: Routledge.

Cooper, A.J. (1892). *A voice from the south*. Xenia, OH: Aldine.

Crenshaw, K. (1991). Mapping the margins: Intersectionality, identity politics, and violence against women of color. *Stanford Law Review*, 43, 1241–1299.

Crenshaw, K. (2003). Traffic at the crossroads: multiple oppressions. (pp. 43–57). In R. Morgan (Ed.). *Sisterhood is forever: The women's anthology for a new millennium*. New York, NY: Washington Square Press.

Crenshaw, K. (2011). Postscript. (pp. 221–234). In H. Lutz, MTH. Vivar and L. Supik (Eds). *Framing Intersectionality: Debates on a multi-faceted concept in gender studies*. Farnham, UK: Ashgate.

Davis, A. (1971). *If they come in the morning: Voices of resistance*. New York, NY: Third Press.

Davis, K. (2008). Intersectionality as buzzword: A sociology of science perspective on what makes a feminist theory successful. *Feminist Theory*, 9(1), 67–85.

De Beauvoir, S. (1984). *The second sex*. Harmondsworth, UK: Penguin Books.

Dhamoon, R. (2011). Considerations on mainstreaming intersectionality. *Political Research Quarterly*, 64(1), 230–243.

Ehrenreich, N. (2002). Subordination and symbiosis: Mechanisms of mutual support between subordinating systems. *University of Missouri-Kansas City Law Review*, 71, 251–324.

Fawcett, B., Featherstone, B., Fook, J. and Rossiter, A. (Eds) (2000). *Practice and research in social work: Postmodern feminist perspectives*. London: Routledge.

Ferree, M. (2009). Inequality, intersectionality and the politics of discourse: Framing feminist alliances. (pp. 86–104). In E. Lombardo, P. Meier and M. Verloo (Eds). *The discursive politics of gender equality: Stretching, bending and policymaking*. London and New York, NY: Routledge.

Fraser, N. (1989). Talking about needs: Interpretive contests as political conflicts in welfare-state societies. *Ethics*, 99(2), 291–313.

Gressgård, R. (2008). Mind the gap: Intersectionality, complexity and 'the event'. *Theory and Science*, 10, 1–16.

Hancock, A.M. (2007). When multiplication doesn't equal quick addition: Examining intersectionality as a research paradigm. *Perspectives on Politics*, 5(1), 63–78.

Haraway, D. (1988). Situated knowledges: The science question in feminism and the privilege of partial perspective. Feminist Studies, 14(3), 575–599.

Haraway, D. (1991). *Simians, cyborgs and women: The reinvention of nature*. London: Free Association Books.

Haraway, D. (1997). *Modest witness@second millenium: FemaleMan meets OncoMouse: Feminism and technoscience*. New York, NY: Routledge.

Haraway, D. (2004). *The Haraway reader*. New York, NY: Routledge.

hooks, b. (1990). *Yearning: Race, gender and cultural politics*. Boston, MA: South End Press.

hooks, b. (2000). *Feminist theory: From margins to center*. Boston, MA: South End Press.

Hopper, K. (1989). Deviance and dwelling space: Notes on the resettlement of homeless persons with alcohol and drug problems. *Contemporary Drug Problems*, 16, 391–414.

Horsell, C. (2006). Homelessness and social exclusion: A Foucauldian perspective for social workers. *Australian Social Work*, 59(2), 213–225.

Hulko, W. (2015). Operationalizing intersectionality in feminist social work research. Reflections and techniques from research with equity-seeking groups (pp. 69–89). In: S. Wahab, B. Anderson-Nathe and C. Gringeri (Eds). *Feminisms in Social Work Research*. New York, NY: Routledge.

Hutchinson, D. (2001). Identity Crisis: Intersectionality, multidimensionality, and the development of an adequate theory of subordination. *Michigan Journal of Race and Law*, 6(2), 285–317.

International Federation of Social Workers. (2005). *Ethics in social work: Statement of principles*. Accessed 12 March 2012. http://ifsw.org/policies/code-of-ethics/.

Jackson, S. and Scott, S. (2010). *Theorising sexuality*. Maidenhead, UK: McGraw-Hill Education.

Jencks, C. (1994). *The homeless*. Cambridge, MA: Harvard University Press.

Johnson, A.K. (1995). Homelessness. In *Encyclopedia of social work* (19th ed.) (pp. 1338–1346). Washington, DC: National Association of Social Workers Press.

Johnson. A.K. and Cnaan, R.A. (1995). Social work practice with homeless persons: State of the art. *Research on Social Work Practice*, 5(3), 340–382.

Johnson, G., Gronda, H. and Coutts, S. (2008). *On the outside: Pathways in and out of homelessness*. Melbourne, Vic: Australian Scholarly Publishing.

Kemp, S. and Brandwein, R. (2010). Feminisms and social work in the United States: An intertwined history. *Affilia: Journal of Women and Social Work*, 25(4), 341–364.

King, D.K. (1988). Multiple jeopardy, multiple consciousness: The context of a black feminist ideology. *Signs: Journal of Women in Culture and Society*, 14(1), 42–72.

Lykke, N. (2010). *Feminist studies: A guide to intersectional theory, methodology, and writing*. New York, NY: Routledge.

McCall, L. (2005). The complexity of intersectionality. *Signs: Journal of Women in Culture and Society*, 30(3), 1771–1800.

McCall, L. (2009). The complexity of intersectionality. (pp. 49–76). In E. Grabham, D. Cooper, J. Krishnadas, and D. Herman (Eds). *Intersectionality and beyond: Law, power and the politics of location*. New York, NY: Routledge-Cavendish.

McKibbin, G., Duncan, R., Hamilton, B., Humphreys, C. and Kellett, C. (2015).The intersectional turn in feminist theory: A response to Carbin and Edenheim (2013). *European Journal of Women's Studies*, 22(1) 99–103.

Matsuda, M. (1991). Beside my sister, facing the enemy: Legal theory out of coalition. *Stanford Law Review*, 43, 1183–1189.

Matsuda, M. (1992). When the first quail calls: Multiple consciousness as jurisprudential method. Women's Rights Law Reporter, 14, 297–300.

Mattsson, T. (2014). Intersectionality as a useful tool: Anti-oppressive social work and critical reflection. *Affilia: Journal of Women and Social Work*, 29(1), 8–17.

May, V.M. (2015). *Pursuing intersectionality: unsettling* dominant imaginaries. New York, NY: Routledge.

Mehrotra, G. (2010). Toward a continuum of intersectionality theorizing for feminist social work scholarship, *Affilia: Journal of Women and Social Work*, 25(4), 417–430.

Minh-ha, Trinh T. (1986). She: The inappropriated other. *Discourse*, 8, 11–37.

Mohanty, C.T. (2003). *Feminism without borders: Decolonizing theory, practicing solidarity*. Durham, NC: Duke University Press.

Mostowska, M. (2014). 'We shouldn't but we do…': Framing the strategies for helping homeless EU migrants in Copenhagen and Dublin. *British Journal of Social Work*, 44(1),18–34.

Murphy, Y., Hunt, V., Zajicek, A.M., Norris, A.N. and Hamilton, L. (2009). *Incorporating intersectionality in social work practice, research, policy, and education*. NASW Press.

Nash, J. (2008). Re thinking intersectionality. *Feminist Review*, 89, 1–15.

National Association of Social Workers (NASW). (2008). *Code of ethics*. Accessed 12 March 2012. www.socialworkers.org/pubs/code/code.asp.

Neale, J. (1997). Homelessness and theory reconsidered. *Housing Studies*, 12(1), 47–61.

Nixon, J. and Humphreys, C. (2010). Marshalling the evidence: Using intersectionality in the domestic violence frame. *Social Politics*, 17(2), 137–158.

Nordfeldt, M. (2012). A dynamic perspective on homelessness: Homeless families in Stockholm. *European Journal of Homelessness*, 6(1), 105–123.

Passaro, J. (1996. Reprint 2014). *The unequal homeless: Men on the streets, women in their place*. London: Routledge.

Pease, B. (2010). *Undoing privilege: Unearned advantage in a divided world*. London: Zed Books.

Phoenix, A. and Pattynama, P. (2006). Editorial: Intersectionality. *European Journal of Women's Studies*, 13(3), 187–192.

Pleace, N. (2000). The new consensus, the old consensus and the provision of services for people sleeping rough. *Housing Studies*, 15(4), 581–594.

Prins, B. (2006). Narrative accounts of origins: A blind spot in the intersectional approach. *European Journal of Women's Studies. Special Issue on Intersectionality*, 13(3), 277–290.

Rosenthal, R. (2000). Imaging homelessness and homeless people: Visions and strategies within the movement. *Journal of Social Distress and the Homeless*, 9(2), 111–126.

Rossi, P.H. (1989). *Down and out in America: The origins of homelessness*. Chicago, IL: University of Chicago Press.

Rowntree, M. (2014). Making sexuality visible in Australian social work education. *Social Work Education*, 33(3), 353–364.

Samuels, M. and Ross-Sheriff, F. (2008). Editorial. Identity, oppression, and power: Feminisms and intersectionality theory. *Affilia: Journal of Women and Social Work*, 23(1), 5–9.

Sandberg, L. (2013). Backward, dumb, and violent hillbillies? Rural geographies and intersectional studies on intimate partner violence. *Affilia: Journal of Women and Social Work*, 28(4) 350–365.

Somerville, P. (1992). Homelessness and the meaning of home: Rooflessness or Rootlessness? *International Journal of Urban and Regional Research*, 16(4), 529–538.

Somerville, P. (2013). Understanding homelessness. *Housing, Theory and Society*, 30(4), 384–415.

Staunaes, D. (2003). Where have all the subjects gone? Bringing together the concepts of intersectionality and subjectification. *NORA Nordic Journal of Women's Studies*, 11(3), 1–10.

Homelessness and social work

38   *Homelessness and social work*

s, S., Walby, S. and Armstrong, J. (2013). Intersectionality and multiplen British policy on violence against women. *Social Politics*,81.
Thornton Dill, B. and Kohlman, M.H. (2012). Intersectionality. (pp. 154–171). In
S. Hesse-Biber (Ed.). *Handbook of feminist research*. Los Angeles, CA: Sage.
Valdes, F. (1995). Sex and race in queer legal culture: Ruminations on identities and
inter-connectivities. (pp. 334–339). In R. Delgado and J. Stefancic (Eds). *Critical race theory: The cutting edge*. Philadelphia, PA: Temple University Press.
Verloo, M. (2006). Multiple inequalities, intersectionality and the European Union. *European Journal of Women's Studies*, 13(3): 211–228.
Wahab, S., Anderson-Nathe, B. and Gringeri, C. (Eds). (2015). *Feminisms in social work research*. New York, NY: Routledge.
Walby, S. (2007). Complexity theory, systems theory and multiple intersecting social inequalities. *Philosophy of the Social Sciences*, 37(4), 449–470.
Weedon, C. (1987). *Feminist practice and poststructuralist theory*. Oxford, UK: Blackwell.
Wendt, S. and Moulding, N. (Eds). (2016). *Contemporary feminisms in social work practice*. Abingdon, UK: Routledge.
Wetherell, M. (1998). Positioning and interpretative repertoire: Conversations analysis and poststructuralism in dialogue. *Discourse and Society*, 9(3), 387–412.
Wilson, A.R. (2013). *The politics of intersectionality. Situating intersectionality: Politics, policy and power*. New York, NY: Palgrave Macmillan.
Wing, A.K. (1990–1991). Brief reflections towards a multiplicative theory and praxis of being. *Berkeley Women's Law Journal*, 6, 181–201.
Winker, G. and Degele, N. (2011). Intersectionality as multi-level analysis: Dealing with social inequality. *European Journal of Women's Studies*, 18(1), 51–66.
Young, I.M. (2011). Five faces of oppression. (pp. 39–66). In *Justice and the Politics of Difference*. Princeton, NJ: Princeton University Press.
Yuval-Davis, N. (2006). Intersectionality and feminist politics. *European Journal of Women's Studies*, 13(3), 193–209.
Yuval-Davis, N. (2011). *Power, intersectionality and the politics of belonging*. FREIA – Feminist Research Center in Aalborg, Aalborg University, Denmark, FREIA Working Paper Series, Working paper no. 75.
Yuval-Davis, N. (2012). Dialogical epistemology: An intersectional resistance to the 'Oppression Olympics.' *Gender and Society*, 26, 46–64.
Yuval-Davis, N. (2015). Situated intersectionality and social inequality. *La Revue Raisons Politiques*, 58, 91–100.
Zufferey, C. (2008). Responses to homelessness in Australian cities: Social worker perspectives. *Australian Social Work*, 61(4), 357–371.
Zufferey, C. (2009). Making gender visible: Social work responses to homelessness. *Affilia: Journal of Women and Social Work*, 24(4), 382–393.
Zufferey, C. (2012). Jack of all trades, master of none? Social work identity and homelessness in Australian cities. *Journal of Social Work*, 12(5), 510–527.
Zufferey, C. (2015). Intersectional feminism and social work responses to homelessness. (pp. 90–103). In S. Wahab, B. Anderson-Nathe and C. Gringeri (Eds). *Feminisms in social work research*. New York, NY: Routledge.
Zufferey, C. (2016). Homelessness and intersectional feminist practice. (pp. 238–249). In S. Wendt and N. Moulding (Eds). *Contemporary feminisms in social work practice*. Abingdon, UK: Routledge.

Zufferey, C. and Chung, D. (2006). Representations of homelessness in the Australian print media: Some implications for social policy. *Just Policy*, 42, 33–38.

Zufferey, C. and Chung, D. (2015). 'Red dust homelessness': housing, home and homelessness in remote Australia. *Journal of Rural Studies*, 41, 13–22.

Zufferey, C. and Kerr, L. (2004). Identity and everyday experiences of homelessness: Some implications for social work. *Australian Social Work*, 57(4), 343–353.

3   Social work research and homelessness

This chapter critically examines research literature in the fields of social work, homelessness and intersectionality. I begin the chapter by locating homelessness literature in social work journals from the USA, UK, Australia and European Union that have drawn on aspects of intersectionality, followed by a discussion of multidisciplinary literature. As there is a dearth of social work literature on homelessness that engages with intersectionality, I highlight my own recent Australian intersectional research projects that explore experiences of home and homelessness. I advocate for further social work research that centralises intersectionality and argue that intersectional social work research can contribute to constructing more complex and dynamic understandings of social work responses to homelessness.

Background

There is a burgeoning amount of research literature in the area of homelessness, particularly from the USA, Canada, UK and Australia. Even in the 1990s, Johnson and Cnaan (1995, p. 361) concluded that in North America 'homelessness is one of the most studied social problems in the last decade'. However, despite attempts to count numbers, construct definitions, examine causes and calculate costs, homelessness is considerably diverse and difficult to enumerate and measure (Jencks, 1994; Johnson, 1995; Williams and Cheal, 2001). Early social science and sociological research on homelessness emerged from the American context, focusing on marginalised and disaffiliated social groups, such as 'hobos' living in skid row areas, often in inner city locations (Anderson, 1923) and later, documented activist social movements and social protests in the field of homelessness (Wright, 1997). UK and Australian policy scholars have particularly advocated a critical, social constructionist approach to homelessness that combines structural and individual explanations and solutions to homelessness, focusing on different pathways for entering and exiting homelessness (Hutson and Clapham, 1999; Pleace, 2000; Clapham, 2005; Johnson *et al.*, 2008). In this chapter, I discuss social work literature on homelessness and intersectionality and multidisciplinary literature on homelessness from different countries. Finally, I discuss my own intersectional research on home and homelessness.

Social work research, homelessness and intersectionality

To obtain a general indication of the engagement of social work literature with homelessness and intersectionality, I completed an online search of key social work journals from the US, UK, Europe and Australia, using the terms 'homeless' and 'intersectionality' (including book reviews, editorials and opinion pieces). From their inceptions, the social work journals have published research on homelessness. However, intersectionality was less common. For example, in America, *Social Work (Journal of the National Association of Social Workers)* (1959–2015) published 370 articles that mentioned the word 'homeless', with ten articles mentioning intersectionality. One practice article focused on domestic violence fatality reviews, intersectionality and homeless services (Chanmugam, 2014). In the journal *Research on Social Work Practice* (1991–2015) I found 163 articles mentioning 'homeless', with nine using the term intersectionality. One article on black men's mental health referred to homelessness and intersectionality (Watkins *et al.*, 2015). Finally, *Affilia: Journal of Women and Social Work* (1986–2015) published the highest number of articles mentioning 'intersectionality' at 112 articles (mostly in the 2000s), and over 160 articles that mentioned the word 'homeless'. In Britain, the *British Journal of Social Work (Journal of the British Association of Social Workers)* (1971–2015) published 314 articles mentioning the word 'homeless', with 33 containing the word 'intersectionality'. Two journal articles discussed an intersectional analysis of the experiences of refugee mothers and South Asian women facing domestic violence and also mentioned homelessness (Anitha, 2010; Vervliet *et al.*, 2014). The *Journal of Social Work* (2001–2015) published 51 articles with the word 'homeless', with six using the term 'intersectionality'. One article on discourses about girls in Israel included brief references to intersectionality and homelessness (Krumer-Nevo *et al.*, 2015). In Australia, *Australian Social Work (Journal of the Australian Association of Social Workers)* (1948–2015) published 230 articles with the term 'homeless' and four with the word 'intersectionality'. Social work education journals were also searched. For example, the UK journal *Social Work Education* (1981–2015) published 136 articles with the term 'homeless' and 24 with the term 'intersectionality' and three articles that mentioned both. As well, *Advances in Social Work and Welfare Education (Australian and New Zealand Social Work and Welfare Education and Research Journal)* was included on the Informit data base in 2011, and since then, one article has been published on homelessness, which did not contain the term 'intersectional' (Horsell, 2013). In 2009, I also wrote a paper on teaching about homelessness and children in this journal (Zufferey, 2009b) but this was before it went online in 2011, and I also did not mention intersectionality. In Europe, the *European Journal of Social Work* (1998–2016) had over 120 articles with the term 'homeless' and five articles that mentioned intersectionality (mostly from 2010 onwards). Two articles mentioned both. Graham and Schiele (2010) compared the equality-of-oppressions paradigm in the USA and the anti-discriminatory framework in the UK, and argued that there has been a declining emphasis on racism in contemporary social work education. In Denmark, Bak and Larsen (2015, p. 15) conducted an inter-categorical quantitative analysis to compare the 'cumulative disadvantage' and poverty individualisation theses, and found that 'class-based explanations and explanations of the individualisation of poverty are less useful than the intersection between structural positions and individual biographies'.

This brief search of key social work journals does indicate that social work literature has historically engaged with homelessness and, more recently, with intersectionality. Intersectional approaches have emerged particularly in social work feminist literature (such as in *Affilia*). Intersectionality is also a recent entry in the *Encyclopaedia of Social Work* (Yamada *et al.*, 2015). However, there is a dearth of articles on intersectional approaches to homelessness in social work literature. In general, social work literature on homelessness has tended to examine and provide evidence for improvements in system and service delivery practices and policies. Further research drawing on intersectional social work approaches would contribute to this literature, by emphasising the intersecting complexities and diversities that constitute the social inequalities of homelessness.

Recently, in the *British Journal of Social Work*, Manthorpe *et al.* (2015, p. 587) called for the social work profession to 'articulate more clearly the potential for social work support to improve outcomes' for people at risk of or experiencing homelessness. Homelessness cannot be avoided in social work practice with 'at risk' young people, children, families and adults (Manthorpe *et al.*, 2015). In the UK, social work research literature on homelessness has tended to be qualitative, such as gathering young homeless people's perspectives of care (De Winter and Noom, 2003), and examining the spatialised politics of belonging for racialised homeless young people (Crath, 2012). Australian social work articles also tended to be qualitative, addressing the following neglected categories and vulnerable groups: pregnant homeless young women (Bessant, 2003), women and violence (Murray, 2011), homeless men (Roche, 2015), homeless fathers (McArthur *et al.*, 2006), homeless 'careers' and pathways such as youth, housing or family breakdown (Chamberlain and Mackenzie, 2006), and older people and homelessness (Lipmann, 2009). Homelessness research has frequently examined a particular homelessness 'characteristic', such as drug and alcohol addictions (see Johnson and Chamberlain, 2008) or mental illness. As well, with the introduction of social inclusion/exclusion policies in Europe, the UK and Australia, social exclusion and homelessness is increasingly being analysed (Kennett and Marsh, 1999; Anderson, 2003; Horsell, 2006; 2014).

When theorising social policy, homelessness and social work researchers have played a role in critically examining political trends, such as social inclusion/exclusion policy discourses (Horsell, 2006). In Europe, Belgian authors in social welfare studies Maeseele *et al.* (2014) examined historical shifts in changing responses to homelessness. They found that the welfare approach to 'vagrancy' was reconstructed as responding to the social problem of homelessness. They also found that the conceptual shift from the criminal problem of vagrancy to homelessness as a poverty problem was 'accompanied by an emphasis on a psycho-social approach to homelessness' (Maeseele *et al.*, 2014, p. 1717). Similar to other European countries, social workers in Flanders (the Dutch speaking part of Belgium) have a mandate to intervene in homelessness. However, according to Maeseele *et al.* (2014, p. 1717) social work responses to homelessness are 'made increasingly conditional' because of the tightening 'accessibility of social services for homeless people'.

Social work journals included articles about social work methods of practice in the field of homelessness by authors from different countries, such as outreaching to 'rough sleepers' in Australia (Parsell, 2011), and the role of social work in 'streetwork' from Israel (Szeintuch, 2015). These journal articles presented evaluations of a practice approach, such as case management with young people (Grace and Gill, 2014), of a service, such as accommodation services (McLaughlin, 2011) and day centres as sanctuaries for the 'undeserving' (Bowpitt *et al.*, 2014, p. 1251). Occasionally, social workers examined neglected geographical locations, such as global/local or urban/rural issues (Sandberg, 2013). In the European Union, there has been a recent emphasis on 'internal' migrants who are experiencing homelessness (Fitzpatrick *et al.*, 2012; Mostowska, 2014).

Intersectionality has been taken up by feminist social work scholars, in particular. The search for the words 'intersectionality', 'intersectional' and 'intersect' in the feminist journal *Affilia* with the SAGE database (1986–2015) yielded over 200 articles (including book reviews and editorials), the largest number in social work journal articles. Of these, eight articles mentioned both 'homeless' and 'intersection' but the topics were diverse and the research did not necessarily use intersectionality as a frame or for an analysis.

Qualitative research articles in *Affilia* that mentioned intersectionality and homelessness included research with social workers, and with women 'at risk' of experiencing homelessness (Zufferey, 2009a; Broussard *et al.*, 2012; Rich, 2014). My article, on how social workers' bodies and identities are gendered, classed and racialised when responding to homelessness, is discussed further in Chapter 5. Two other research articles made visible the experiences of women who lived with a disability, in poverty, with intimate partner violence and were at risk of homelessness (Broussard *et al.*, 2012; Rich, 2014). Homelessness was mentioned in narrative research interviews with 19 women with disabilities who experienced intimate partner violence (Rich, 2014). In this study, American social worker Karen Rich (2014, p. 418) intersected gender, victimisation and disability discourses that shaped women's perceptions of IPV, and found that these 'accounts tended to bolster a stereotypically feminine (gendered, nurturant, or sexual) identity'. In another study on the coping skills of 12 poor women who raised their children alone, their experiences of and increasing risk of abuse and homelessness was mentioned briefly (Broussard *et al.*, 2012). These qualitative analyses of narrative interviews were consistent with Danish sociologists Christensen and Jensen's (2012, p. 144) suggestions, that a life story narrative analysis is useful to capture intersections in social structures and institutions, and to show how social identity categories (or locations) intersect in the 'discursive construction of meaning'.

Few quantitative studies were found in the feminist social work journal *Affilia* that mentioned the words 'homeless' and 'intersection'. One article examined associations between depression and three forms of intimate partner violence – economic, physical/sexual and emotional abuse (Voth Schrag, 2015), using data from 3,282 women with children, interviewed in waves 4 and 5 of the Fragile Families and Child Wellbeing Study (Voth Schrag, 2015). It found that economic and physical abuse was partially mediated by depression and had strong correlations with later experiences of material hardship, including homelessness (Voth Schrag, 2015). The researcher argued that intimate partner violence advocates (such as social workers) would do well to consider the added risks associated with economic abuse intersecting with racism, sexism, classism, poverty and other structural inequalities (Voth Schrag, 2015, p. 350). One further article examined ambivalent sexism theory and abortion attitudes, intersecting socio-demographic categories according to religion, age, gender and race/ethnicity (Begun and Walls, 2015) – but this article did not identify homelessness except in one author's biography. Experimental quantitative studies (such as randomised control trials) are not common in social work literature on homeless population groups, as they are often transient and difficult to locate.

One mixed-method study published in *Affilia* that mentioned 'intersection' and 'homeless' researched female heads of households who relied on welfare, and the multilayered barriers they faced in their attempts to obtain employment (Bowie and Dopwell, 2013). This study documented the oppressive racialised and gendered experiences of 30 female respondents, aged 25–34, who were of African American and Latino background (Bowie and Dopwell, 2013, p. 190) using intersectionality. In the USA, in 2007, African Americans and Latinos constituted 12.6 per cent and 16.3 per cent of the population, respectively – but they accounted for 35.5 per cent and 27 per cent of the 1.7 million accessing 'Temporary Assistance for Needy Families' (TANF) (Bowie and Dopwell, 2013). This journal article is further discussed in more detail in the policy chapter, Chapter 4.

Two further articles examined the constructions of policy programmes and the design and delivery of services (Goodkind, 2005; Kennedy, 2008). For example, Goodkind (2005) reviewed assumptions about the increasing numbers of girls in the juvenile justice system and provided a feminist critique of how service responses essentialise gender, reify categories of gender, race, class and sexuality and reinforce gendered norms, therefore locating problems within individuals (not structures) and focusing on girls' victimisation and punishment (Goodkind, 2005, p. 52). As well, Kennedy (2008) provides a history of social workers' responses to young women and eugenics (improving genetics) by examining issues of gender, race, ethnicity and class simultaneously. However, homelessness and/or intersections are mentioned only briefly in these articles. Whilst Broussard *et al.* (2012) and Bowie and Dopwell (2013) explored female-headed households living in poverty (some who experienced homelessness and substandard housing), and Zufferey (2009) examined social work responses to homelessness, none of these articles specifically researched intersecting power relations, in regard to the perspectives of people who experienced 'homelessness'. Therefore, I conclude that previous social work research does not emphasise homelessness and intersectionality (or intersectional feminism), and that the experiences of people affected by homelessness require further attention.

In the *Journal of Poverty*, Norris *et al.* (2010) explored poverty research in rural areas. They argued that an intersectional perspective would make visible 'the complexity of people's social locations by conceptualizing race, class, gender as simultaneously interacting power relations' (Norris *et al.*, 2010, p. 55). They observe that there are:

> Three tendencies in rural poverty scholarship: (a) a tendency to acknowledge the importance of race, gender, or age in shaping rural poverty; (b) a tendency to separate race, gender, and age; and (c) a tendency to treat them as descriptive variables and not as power relationships.
>
> (Norris *et al.*, 2010, p. 57)

This article makes a case for examining poverty from an intersectional perspective that acknowledges power relations – but it does not discuss homelessness and social work in depth, except by implication.

Multidisciplinary literature on homelessness in the USA, UK and Europe

As previously noted, research literature on homelessness has different emphases in different countries (Fitzpatrick and Christian, 2006), with a changing emphasis over time. The USA has the largest research literature on homelessness in the English-speaking world, with Britain second. In 2003, the *Journal of Community and Applied Psychology* published a Special Issue on *Homelessness: Integrating International Perspectives*, edited by Julie Christian and Isobel Anderson, who argued that 'psychology together with other disciplines such as sociology, geography and policy studies can be complementary in meeting the challenges of researching, evaluating and understanding the issues' (Christian, 2003, p. 85). However, as evident in this quote, social work was not included as a discipline that can contribute to researching homelessness.

In Britain, social policy authors in housing studies tended to dominate academic research on housing and homelessness policy (Burrows *et al.*, 1997; Kennett and Marsh, 1999; Pleace, 2000; Anderson, 2003), including social exclusion (Kennett and Marsh, 1999). Social policy literature on homelessness has focused on key policy and legislation changes, including the decriminalisation of vagrancy, deinstitutionalisation policies and changing housing and welfare policies (Kennett and Marsh, 1999; Jones, 2013). Homelessness literature has included social relations related to class, gender (Watson and Austerberry, 1986; Doherty, 2001) and race (Harrison, 1999). In the 1990s, UK academics covering homelessness were in the fields of health (Klee and Reid, 1998), sociology and ex-service men (Higate, 1997), criminology (Carlen, 1996) and socio-legal studies (Cowan, 1999). By the 1990s, homelessness was also beginning to be theorised as a multi-dimensional, social construct (Somerville, 1992; Hutson and Liddiard, 1994; Jacobs *et al.*, 1999). However, social work was generally not considered in this literature.

In the EU, The European Observatory on Homelessness was founded by the European Federation of European Organisations Working with the Homeless (FEANTSA) to conduct transnational research on homelessness and housing exclusion. More recently, research collaborations between housing scholars in the UK and other countries in the EU are common (Doherty *et al.*, 2004; O'Sullivan *et al.*, 2010). As well, the connection between internal and global migration and homelessness is of increasing concern in UK and EU literature (Pleace, 2010). As discussed in the next chapter, few European authors such as Bezunartea-Barrio (2014) and Benjaminsen (2014) have explored the changing roles of social workers in a changing European social and political context.

In the USA, homelessness has been researched in anthropological and sociological studies (Snow and Anderson, 1987; Wright, 1988; Wright, 1997; Wright and Rubin, 1991), economics (Quigley *et al.*, 2001), as well as social science, law and psychology (Rossi, 1989a; 1989b; Blasi, 1990). In America, the term 'homeless' was not widely used until the late 1970s when social advocate Mitch Snyder argued that millions of Americans were homeless (Jencks, 1994, p. 1). Traditionally, literature in the field of homelessness focused on individual characteristics and economic inequalities, such as poverty (Blau, 1992), deviancy, class relations, and men in 'skid row' hotels, particularly highlighting alcohol abuse (Rossi, 1989a; 1989b; Jencks, 1994). Psychological and medical perspectives have tended to dominate homeless research (Shinn and Weitzman, 1990). This prominence may be linked to welfare provision arrangements, where health-oriented responses and disciplines are common.

Quantitative studies have also dominated the US research landscape on homelessness, examining differences (such as age, gender and race) as descriptive variables (Norris *et al.*, 2010). Canadian sociologist and social development scholar Peressini (2009, p. 13) quantitatively tested the heterogeneous hypothesis of homelessness, by examining age, gender, marital status, ethnicity and education, and found that 'homelessness due to poverty, interpersonal conflict, health, and addictions vary considerably by age, while gender affects the likelihood of reporting interpersonal conflict, health problems, and housing issues'. Whilst these inter-categorical studies are useful for understanding how social discriminations contribute to homelessness, quantitative studies tend not to discuss micro–macro power relation and intersecting social inequalities in great depth.

Dating back to the 1980s, there has been considerable work undertaken by US social policy researchers, such as Dennis Culhane and colleagues at the University of Pennsylvania, on costing supportive housing, as well as programme evaluations for people who experience chronic homelessness, mental illness, health issues and disabilities, including veterans and at-risk children and families (Culhane *et al.*, 2002; Culhane, 2008). Moreover, there have been numerous quantitative and qualitative evaluations of Housing First services for people who experience homelessness, with co-occurring serious mental illness and substance abuse (Padgett *et al.*, 2006). As discussed in the next chapter (Chapter 4), particularly since the introduction of Housing First initiatives, the changing role and 'treatment first' 'mindset' of social workers in responding to homelessness has been taken up in the European context (Benjaminsen, 2014, p. 12). Social work authors such as Benjaminsen (2014) argue that Housing First is a social justice and human rights issue for people who experience homelessness and that this approach resonates with social work ethics and values. However, I note that these studies have not attended to or incorporated intersectionality.

In contrast to the USA, the welfare state in Britain has tended to fund smaller social policy-oriented research (Fitzpatrick and Christian, 2006). British research on homelessness has drawn upon interpretive, social constructionist and critical approaches (Jacobs *et al.*, 1999). This literature has been synthesised by Fitzpatrick and Christian (2006), who argue that there are lessons for each country. For example, they report that Britain needs more robust quantitative longitudinal research with careful sampling and comparisons groups, whilst the USA needs more critical reflection, qualitative and policy impact research (Fitzpatrick and Christian, 2006). Whilst there is some resistance to psychological approaches within British social policy research, due to concerns about 'individualising' social problems and 'pathologising' disadvantaged groups, Fitzpatrick and Christian (2006, p. 325) argue that these studies can provide insights into individual cognition, emotion and motivation. The disciplinary backgrounds of researchers inevitably shape how research on homelessness is constructed, with implications for how intersectionality is used (or not).

Furthermore, Bacchi (2009) examined the role played by academic researchers in the processes of knowledge production and the relationship between researchers and policy makers. She makes a strong case for all researchers (including social workers), to pay greater critical attention to the effects of the evidence-based policy paradigm. Social workers engaged in policy research are often positioned as 'social scientists' that are simply delivering 'evidence' on questions and priorities set by governments, espe-cially if the research is funded by governments. This positioning makes it difficult to subject policy priorities and problem representations to scru-tiny, and to reflect more broadly on their implications (Bacchi, 2009), and their unintended consequences.

Homelessness research (particularly in the British context but also in Australia) has been criticised for becoming too closely aligned with pol-icy funding and agendas, shaping the construction of 'special' categories of homelessness, such as young people, rough sleepers, women and older people (Pleace and Quilgars, 2003). This research then informs policy pro-cesses about 'homeless pathways', including mental health, domestic vio-lence, housing crises, substance abuse and youth pathways (Johnson *et al.*, 2008). However, as discussed in Chapter 5, the gendered, sexualised, racial-ised and classed power relations inherent in institutionalised practices and the categorisation of client identities, and managerialist approaches (such as case management) in social work organisations can create ethical dilem-mas for social workers in the field of homelessness (Horsell, 2006; Zufferey, 2008).

Lastly, homelessness and social work research and literature has been dominated by individual and/or structural debates (Pleace and Quilgars, 2003; Chamberlain *et al.*, 2014). Individual risk factors, or 'characteristics' of people who are defined as homeless, are constructed as being associated with poverty, having disabilities, abusing drugs and alcohol, experiencing mental illness, emotional and psychological distress, low levels of educa-tion, limited employment options and engaging in criminal activity. Whilst research has examined structural causes of homelessness, people who experience homelessness are often perceived and responded to within an 'individual sickness' paradigm (Wasserman and Clair, 2010, p. 8). Structural explanations of homelessness have included deinstitutionalisation policies, changes in the labour market, declining affordable housing options, chang-ing family structures and low wages. As well, economic inequalities, patri-archal systems and gendered citizenship have been associated with domestic and family violence contributing to women's homelessness (Zufferey *et al.*, 2016). Social workers have combined structural and individual consid-erations in their engagement with the social justice values of social work, which informs their activist responses to homelessness (Zufferey, 2008). However, Wasserman and Clair (2010) have argued that this individualist-structural debate misses the mark on key concerns for people who are actu-ally experiencing homelessness. As further discussed in Chapter 6, I centre the perspectives of diverse groups of people who experience homelessness, consistent with a social work and intersectional commitment to the pursuit of social justice. In this book I posit that intersectional social work research can emphasise both structural and individual or macro and micro power relations, by examining intersecting social processes and political institu-tions that continue to shape social inequalities.

Gender and race relations

Although not all in social work, there is also considerable historical and contemporary literature in the area of women's homelessness. This has included: researching characteristics of homeless women (Johnson and Kreuger, 1989) and homeless families (Johnson, 1989; Stewart and Steward, 1992; Shinn and Weitzman, 1996), advocating for strengths and feminist approaches to women's homelessness (Johnson and Richards, 1995; Boes and van Wormer, 1997), documenting the narratives and lived experiences of 'homeless' women (Williams, 2003; Scott, 2007; Casey *et al.*, 2008) and children (Moore *et al.*, 2011), exploring domestic and childhood violence and homelessness (Nyamathi *et al.*, 1999), exploring the effects of domestic violence on increasing women's risk of homelessness (Murray, 2011), emphasising the role of intimate partner violence in relationships and pathways out of and into homelessness (Williams, 1998; Jones *et al.*, 2012), emphasising survival and sex work (Harding and Hamilton, 2009; Watson, 2011), documenting the difficulties of mothering when homeless (Connolly, 2000; Jasinski *et al.*, 2010), questioning gendered constructs of home and identity (Wardhaugh, 1999) and in policy (Paterson, 2010), examining women's access to housing, trajectories and life histories from a feminist approach (Watson and Austerberry, 1986; Tomas and Dittmar, 1995; Watson, 2000), promoting feminist social work practice in the area of homelessness (Watson and Austerberry, 1986; Johnson and Richards, 1995) and highlighting structural factors such as inequalities in the labour market and the feminisation of poverty (Pearce, 1978; Baptista, 2010). Ethnographic studies in this field have also been common, examining subjective understandings of homelessness, survival strategies and the broader (gendered) political and social aspects of home and homelessness (Russell, 1991; Snow and Anderson, 1993; Liebow, 1995; Passaro, 1996; Wright, 1997; Wardhaugh, 1999). Research drawing on intersectionality has tended to focus on domestic violence (Sokoloff and Dupont, 2005; Nixon and Humphreys, 2010), including domestic violence in social work (Laing and Humphreys, 2013) and women's homelessness in Australia (Martin, 2014). However, these studies that take an intersectional approach have not examined homelessness and social work practices more broadly.

Women's experiences of becoming homeless differ from those of men because they are more likely to be subjected to childhood abuse and intimate partner violence, experience trauma and psychological distress, be the main care provider for children, be living in poverty and use informal supports such as family and friends, before accessing a service or sleeping rough (Zufferey *et al.*, 2016). However, these experiences potentially differ across racial/ethnic groups of women, class, sexuality, ability and geographical location, to name some social markers. Quantitative studies on homelessness have tended to focus on ethnicity, race, gender and economic inequalities as variables in research. However, these studies do not tend to theorise the findings within unequal power relations, using intersectionality. For example, in the

USA, psychologists Nyamathi *et al.* (1999) compared socio-demographic, behavioural, victimisation and psychological differences among 448 homeless women and their male partners in the context of the prevention of Acquired Immune Deficiency Syndrome (AIDS). The majority of the women and their intimate partners in Nyamathi *et al.*'s (1999) study were African American (59 per cent and 65 per cent, respectively); fewer participants were Mexican/Hispanic (23 per cent of women and 24 per cent of men) and Caucasian (17 per cent of women and 10 per cent of men). Men were more likely to be employed (33 per cent) compared to women (12 per cent) (Nyamathi *et al.*, 1999, p. 493). They found that homeless women scored significantly lower on mental health, self-esteem, drug use and significantly higher on depression, anxiety and childhood and adult sexual abuse, than their intimate partners. These studies provide useful knowledge to the field but tend not to be positioned within the radical tradition of intersectionality (May, 2015).

The connection between intimate partner violence (IPV) and women's homelessness has also been well documented (Browne and Bassuk, 1997; Zufferey, 2016). Intimate partner violence is the primary reason for women's homelessness (Chung *et al.*, 2000). Safe and appropriate housing and the economic resources for its maintenance are two of the most pressing concerns for women wanting to escape IPV. Following separation from a violent partner, women and their children are likely to experience significant income loss, financial hardship and housing instability, particularly those who have been at least partially financially dependent on their partners (Pavao *et al.*, 2007; Baker *et al.*, 2009). In the USA, Pavao *et al.*'s (2007, p. 143) quantitative analysis of the California Women's Health Survey conducted in 2003 found that women who experienced IPV in the last year are four times more likely to report housing instability than other women, including late rent or mortgage payments, frequent moves and being without their own housing. As well, Baker *et al.* (2003; 2009; 2010) found that housing problems were worse among women who experienced severe violence, contacted fewer formal systems, had less informational support and had received a negative response from formal welfare services. Women who have been (or are) subjected to IPV encounter multiple systemic barriers to accessing safe and appropriate housing, often placing them and their children at risk of further exposure to IPV (Clough *et al.*, 2014, p. 685). However, when exploring how gender and race intersect, it has been noted that the interaction of individual, familial, social and cultural barriers to help-seeking may differ for women of different cultural backgrounds, such as Latino survivors of IPV (Postmus *et al.*, 2014, p. 464). Intersectionality is used more often in social work research on IPV (rather than homelessness), which points to the feminist origins of IPV theorising.

To analyse gendered inequalities and the effects of IPV on women's housing, mental health, employment and social participation, my Australian colleagues Suzanne Franzway, Donna Chung, Sarah Wendt, Nicole Moulding and I have recently completed a large Australian study,[1] gathering data from

over 600 women in a national online survey (along with 17 in-depth interviews). In this large Australian survey, the majority of the sample reported
that their sexual orientation was heterosexual (94.5 per cent), they were not
currently experiencing IPV (82.4 per cent), they had children (79 per cent) and
they lived in a city or suburban area (65.8 per cent). The majority of respondents were born in Australia (81.2 per cent) and considered their cultural identity to be Australian (78.7 per cent), followed by Northern/Western Europe
(12.2 per cent), with small numbers from the Middle East, Asia/South East
Asia, South America and Africa. Incomes were in the lower ranges, with 40.6
per cent currently earning under A$30,000 per annum. Unlike previous stud-
ies in the US, such as the one by Dewey and Germain (2014, p. 390) in which
the highest income level for women accessing transitional housing services
was US$25,000 annually, 8.1 per cent of the sample in this community-based
study reported an annual income of A$90,000 and over. This level of income
exceeds the average male and female salary in Australia (ABS, 2014). Despite
these earnings, many women (with their children) had to make frequent and
significant geographical moves to escape violence (42 per cent of total survey respondents). The sample of women who responded to the online survey
did not have to identify as experiencing homelessness. However, 1.8 per cent
of women reported living in 'impoverished dwellings' such as cars, streets or
parklands. Also, 33 per cent of survey respondents reported staying with family or friends immediately after leaving their partner/s, with only 10 per cent
using women's shelters. We found that IPV exacerbated women's housing,
mental health, employment and community participation barriers, adversely
affecting their ability to participate in civil society and act as empowered citizens (see Zufferey *et al.*, 2016 for further details).

Particularly in the USA, race and gender discriminations that increase
the risks of persistent homelessness are well documented (Passaro, 2014).
As further discussed in Chapter 6, my Australian research has also aimed to
make visible the perspectives of racially diverse community groups (including Aboriginal Australians), by exploring differing experiences of home and
homelessness (Zufferey and Kerr, 2004; Zufferey and Chung, 2015; Zufferey,
2015). However, American social policy and social work authors Norris
et al. (2010), consider how racial inequality can be subsumed under gender
in intersectional theorising. For example, they discuss how the feminisation
of poverty thesis during the 1990s, which defined the experience of poverty
in relation to gender, made invisible 'the fact that Black women have historically had higher poverty rates than White women' (Norris *et al.*, 2010, p. 63).
Despite researchers in this field espousing social justice commitments, May
(2015) also asserts that intersectionality is frequently used in narrow ways that
depoliticises the concept of intersections.

Furthermore, it is important for intersectional researchers to examine how
oppression and privilege are structurally maintained. For example, historically, white women have been encouraged and expected to stay at home as
economically dependent wives and mothers, while black women have been

encouraged and expected to engage in 'breadwinning activities' (Norris *et al.*, 2010, p. 63). This latter expectation was related to minimum wage laws that did not tend to cover black men and women, and therefore, 'Black women's identities could not be constructed solely in relation to their roles as mothers and wives' (Norris *et al.*, 2010, p. 63). Women from ethnic minority back-grounds, such as African American women or Aboriginal Australian women, continue to be more likely to have children in their care, be poor, experience abuse and violence, be discriminated against in employment and have fewer long-term accommodation options. When intersecting gender and race, Norris *et al.* (2010, pp. 62–63) note that the concept of 'racialised gender' is useful to understand how 'gender ideologies, practices, and expectations operate differently across racial/ethnic groups'. For example, as discussed later in this chapter, home and homelessness can be variously experienced and interpreted. When theorising home, home can feel like a prison for some women who experience violence in their homes – but home can also be a 'haven' from a racist society and a site of resistance to 'white supremacist capitalist patriarchy' (hooks, 1990).

During the 1970s the 'cultural turn' in academic research contributed to deconstructing social processes, emotions, meanings, identities, beliefs and values (Best, 2007). According to Best (2007), by the 1980s there was a bur-geoning focus on cultural studies, identity politics and multiculturalism, in relation to changing social, economic, cultural and political institutions. However, research on homelessness has tended to treat interrelated issues such as class, gender, race, ethnicity, sexuality and geographical location as separate research domains or individual identity categories, without acknowl-edging their intersections.

Intersectionality is contested. However, it provides for a 'resistant imagi-nary' that acknowledges multifaceted subjectivities, as well as the complex and multiple social structures that contribute to oppressing and privileging social practices (May, 2015). An intersectional framework can broaden social work research and activism in the area of homelessness. This can include challenging social processes and identity categorisations, as well as examin-ing geographical, social and economic developmental contexts (Yuval-Davis, 2006; Nixon and Humphreys, 2010). Furthermore, social work researchers who engage in intersectional research on homelessness can examine mutually reinforcing social processes that both oppress and privilege. At the micro-political level, this can include exploring individual subjectivities and diverse lived experiences of homelessness. At the macro level, this can involve exam-ining structural, political, philosophical and representational complexities of homelessness that contribute to maintaining social inequalities and injustices.

Intersectionality is not widely discussed in social work literature, but it is an ideal tool for examining the complexities between and within different popu-lation groups (Murphy *et al.*, 2009). In this book I argue that the individual and/or structural debate in social work literature can be broadened, to incor-porate intersectional theorising in social work and homelessness research.

Yet, the 'doing' of intersectional feminist research is complicated and contested. At a minimum, social work research would include an analysis of two or more categories of identity (or social locations), explaining oppression as well as privilege (Murphy *et al.*, 2009, pp. 52–54; Hulko, 2015). Intersectional research has to be political, intentional and integrated into a theoretical framework that attends to how these differences intersect.

Social work academic Hulko (2015, pp. 77–85) discussed how she operationalised intersectionality in five different social work research projects by: sampling for diversity, asking research participants directly about their social location (for example, 'Does being a [woman, Afro-Cuban, lesbian] make a difference in any way? How?'), facilitating diverse voices through eliciting diverse responses to visual objects such as photographs, as well as disseminating data in collaboration with community members to influence social change. Next, I discuss my own Australian research projects that have drawn on intersectional theorising.

My own 'intersectional type' research

My own research on home and homelessness also aimed to sample for diversity, and consult with different research participants about their meanings of home, using diverse research methods, including reflecting on visual artefacts and feelings of home and homelessness (Zufferey and Rowntree, 2014). Relevant to my studies on home and homelessness is the work of sociologist Yuval-Davis (2011), who theorises intersectionality within the concepts of 'belonging' and 'the politics of belonging'. Belonging involves emotional attachment to 'home/s', whilst the politics of belonging relates to the power involved in constructing social boundaries that include and exclude particular categories of people (Yuval-Davis, 2011, pp. 10–18), such as the housed and the homeless. Belonging is about feeling 'at home' and hoping for a 'safe' place to call home (Ignatieff, 2001). Feelings of disconnection from a sense of 'home' and safety are common for the majority of people who experience homelessness. Homelessness can include migrants and refugees 'feeling at home' (or not) in a new country, as well as feelings of safety (or not) in the 'family home' (Zufferey, 2015). The politics of belonging relate to specific political projects that aim to construct belonging to particular collectivity/ies, in very specific ways, with specific boundaries (Yuval-Davis, 2011, pp. 4–5). This can include researching people's emotions about belonging to particular social collectives, related to, for example, gender, race, ethnicity, culture, sexuality, class, ability, age, mobility, wealth, religion, geographical location, nation state and a country's social and economic developmental contexts (Yuval-Davis, 2006; Nixon and Humphreys, 2010). An intersectional framework around the notion of belonging and the politics of belonging (Yuval Davis, 2011) can broaden the social work political project in the area of home and homelessness.

In three of my recent studies I have used an intersectional approach to examine diverse notions of home and homelessness. The first project gathered the perspectives of Aboriginal and non-Aboriginal service providers about how they conceptualised and responded to homelessness in a remote geographical location (Zufferey and Chung, 2015). In the second project I took a 'majority inclusive' approach to explore understandings of home more broadly across different ages, class backgrounds, migration and refugee experiences (Zufferey, 2015). The third project involved exploring home, gender and sexuality in more depth, using visual artefacts or objects as a prompt for discussing experiences of home and homelessness (Zufferey and Rowntree, 2014).

For the first project, Professor Donna Chung (who is currently working at Curtin University, in Western Australia) and I travelled over 2,000 kms (return) from Perth to two remote mining towns in Western Australia, with the then CEO of a domestic violence service in one of these towns. The aim of this research was to explore how homelessness is defined and responded to in remote geographical locations, in towns with high population numbers of Indigenous Australians. We gathered the perspectives of eight service providers through focus groups (Zufferey and Chung, 2015). Seven of the eight service providers were female and one was male. Service providers were employed in domestic violence services, local government, employment, drug and alcohol, community development and health services. The majority of the service providers had moved to the towns to work. Two participants were of Aboriginal/Indigenous background and could speak from an 'insiders' perspective about issues for Aboriginal people and communities in this Western Australian location. One non-Aboriginal service provider identified as being 'from' the local 'Goldfields' area. The remaining five service providers were from other parts of Australia and other countries. The conversations in the focus groups related to dilemmas in service delivery, funding arrangements, policy definitions and practice responses, when working with Aboriginal families and communities in remote locations. The key findings of this research were that normative policy definitions of homelessness that focused on 'living in a house' as a 'home' were not always culturally relevant for local Aboriginal communities. As well, there was limited access to adequate housing options in both communities. Furthermore, 'top down' funding and decisions often occurred without community consultation, fragmenting service delivery, limiting 'grassroots' participation and constraining opportunities for locally relevant service responses (Zufferey and Chung, 2015, p. 13). Consistent with McCall's (2005) anti-categorical research approach, these findings highlight Westernised and urban assumptions that underpin the policy domain in which housing and homelessness responses are determined, emphasising the limits of current policy conceptualisations and interventions, by making visible the perspectives of service providers working in remote areas.

The second research project undertaken with Dr Tammy Hand used an intersectional approach to examine 'majority inclusive' and diverse notions of home and homelessness in Adelaide, South Australia (Zufferey, 2015). We commenced the research with the assumption that conceptualisations of home and homelessness are relative and complex, influenced by changing gender and power relations and historical, discursive, political and cultural contexts. As Christensen and Jensen (2012, p. 120) argue, life story narratives involve 'taking everyday life as point of departure' and analysing unmarked (invisible) social categories that show differences between and within social groups, thereby highlighting intersecting social categorisations and processes. This study used life story narrative analysis to examine 'the complex process of identification and positioning' and 'discursive construction of meaning' (Christensen and Jensen, 2012, p. 114), by focusing on meanings and material experiences of home and homelessness. We gathered the narratives of three men and ten women of different migration experiences, ethnicities, classes, genders and ages through individual narrative interviews. This research shows how notions of home and homelessness intersect with the influences of class, migration and refugee experiences (Zufferey, 2015). The findings highlighted diverse perspectives on and identifications with home/s (and homelessness) in Australia, relating to the experiences of refugee displacement and migration experiences, as well as to a sense of belonging through class aspirations. More details about the findings of this research are discussed in Chapter 6.

In the third research project with my colleague Dr Margaret Rowntree, we examined the intersections between gender and sexuality, in regard to home and homelessness (Zufferey and Rowntree, 2014). This project was conceptualised after I had previously examined race, gender and class relations, but neglected to sample for sexuality. My colleague whose area of research interest is sexuality questioned my research frame and asked: 'where is sexuality on your axes of difference?' As Rowntree (2014) notes, sexuality is frequently neglected in social work education, research, policy and practice. Certainly, a disproportionate number of young people who experience homelessness identify as being lesbian, gay, bisexual and transgender and are more likely to be discriminated against, bullied and verbally or physically harassed at school and in their family (Cochran *et al.*, 2002; Christiani *et al.*, 2008; Corliss *et al.*, 2011). Consequently, we joined forces to undertake a research project, focusing particularly on gender, sexuality and home/homelessness. We explored how sexuality and notions of home and homelessness are embodied and imagined by asking men and women to reflect on objects or visual artefacts of their choice in individual interviews and focus groups (Zufferey and Rowntree, 2014). Following the works of Kuhn (2007) and Pink (2007) on visual methodologies, we asked research participants to bring along an artefact that represented home or homelessness to them. Visual and auditory objects can 'place' a person within the space and the emotional connections that embed them within 'home' (Gibson, 2004), evoking deeply embodied narratives.

We have published the findings from three face-to-face interviews and a focus group of six women (all over 50 years old) who identified as lesbian (Zufferey and Rowntree, 2014). For this small group of lesbian women, 'home' involved the embodiment (and imagining) of physical spaces and locality (including houses and landscapes) and the identification with communities of shared interest, particularly lesbian communities but also environmental movements. Two men participated in this research but their narratives differed and tended to focus on objects and practices in their house as 'home' and experiences of abuse in their childhood. The two men did not express a sense of belonging to a community or collective as 'home' on the basis of their sexuality. The findings of this study resonated with Pilkey's (2013) work, in which he found that sexual identity is often closeted in the parental home and as adults, 'new homes' provide opportunities for freer sexual expression. Sexuality is mutually articulated with practices associated with ethnicity, migration, poverty, class, religion and nations, in ways that individuals negotiate and remember home places and spaces (Fortier, 2003).

Similar to Hulko's (2015, p. 80) intersectional social work research that used visual methods such as photography to elicit the perspectives of lesbian, bisexual and transgender people, we also found that visual objects were useful to elicit participant's varied recollections. This included multiple lived experiences, meaning constructions and subjective positionings, in relation to imagined and embodied relationships with 'home' (and homelessness). The use of visual artefacts in our research prompted women's and men's recollections of deeply held emotional experiences of home, which varied widely. For example, one woman who experienced homelessness explained how she had constructed living spaces from wooden boxes, in a van in which she lived. These artefacts connected emotionally to individual experiences, histories and identities. This study challenged heteronormative assumptions that influence how home and homelessness are understood by giving 'voice' to more diverse understandings, including a collective sense of belonging to a community based on sexual identification (see Zufferey and Rowntree, 2014 for further details).

My three research projects have highlighted how intersecting social and geographical locations can be explored differently in social work research on home and homelessness. This research has illustrated that an intersectional social work approach to researching homelessness is able to: focus on remote geographical locations to deconstruct urbanised policy constructions of homelessness (akin to anti-categorical research), interview a 'majority inclusive' sample using narrative interviewing techniques about diverse and subjective perceptions of home, and make visible the perspectives of a specific minority population group who identify as lesbian or gay, using creative research methodologies. I also discuss another project on sexuality and age in Chapter 6 (Rowntree and Zufferey, 2015).

Conclusion

There are potentially numerous dilemmas experienced by social workers who plan to engage in intersectional homelessness research, including: which intersecting social categories are privileged, what to focus on in multilayered social work responses to homelessness, how to think simultaneously about structures, dynamics and subjectivities, including the different effects of representations of homelessness, how to design an intersectional research project and to analyse intersectional data.

A dilemma in designing intersectional research is deciding what actual social categories are going to be given attention and why. In retrospect, in my own research, I have tended to focus on commonly examined categories such as, responses to homelessness in rural, remote and urban locations (Zufferey and Chung, 2015; Zufferey, 2015), power, gender and class locations of social work and social workers (Zufferey, 2009), as well as age, class, gender, culture, migration, sexuality and meanings of home (Rowntree and Zufferey, 2014; Zufferey, 2015). Therefore, my research attention has rendered invisible other neglected social categories, such as religion, disability and the geography of places and spaces (McDowell, 1999).

When designing intersectional research, it is important to continually ask ourselves how social workers contribute to privileging and oppressing social processes, making invisible inequalities and constituting who remains marginalised. Research in social work has tended to treat marginalised groups as 'the others', to homogenise their experiences and make invisible in-group complexities 'under the guise of generalisability' (Murphy *et al.*, 2009, p. 36). A further dilemma in intersectional research is that participants may not wish to explicitly define their own 'axes of intersectionality', raising questions about who defines who as oppressed and privileged, and the processes of self-identification (Murphy *et al.*, 2009, p. 55).

As well, whilst I frequently use the terms 'diverse' and 'complex', Gressgård (2008, p. 1) observes that key concepts used in intersectional research such as 'complexity' and 'multiplicity' can actually obscure more than they reveal. It is important for social workers to ask how intersectional analyses can examine intersecting power relations that are mutually constitutive, which includes focusing on identities, dynamics and social processes that constitute social inequalities, without reducing everything to being simply 'multiple' and 'complex'.

A key concept in intersectional social work research is that differences are socially categorised around socially constructed norms and embedded in unequal power relations (Murphy *et al.*, 2009, p. 52). An intersectional analysis is useful for examining how social processes, identity categories/subjectivities and unequal power relations interplay to constitute social work responses to homelessness. Depending on disciplinary and theoretical influences, intersectionality has developed in multiple ways. The classic race/gender/class intersections can be broadened in intersectional research, to include an unlimited range of categories, such as sexuality, disability, religion, age, physical location and diverse other social divisions, including the intersection of gender/sex (Lykke, 2010a; 2010b). Social work researchers using intersectional approaches negotiate this complex terrain to find ways of researching social issues that suit their personal and professional values and the aims of the study they wish to pursue.

In this chapter, I have examined social work literature on homelessness and intersectionality. I have discussed homelessness literature in the USA, UK and Europe, gender and race relations and included my own Australian intersectional research projects. The next chapter explores intersectionality in policy making and analysis, by examining definitions of homelessness in policy and legislation and Housing First initiatives.

Note

1 'Gendered Violence and Citizenship: the complex effects of intimate partner violence on mental health, housing and employment', which is funded by Australian Research Council Project No: DP1130104437.

References

Anderson, I. (2003). Synthesizing homelessness research: Trends, lessons and prospects. *Journal of Community and Applied Social Psychology*, 13, 197–205.

Anderson, N. (1923). *The hobo: The sociology of the homeless man*. Chicago, IL: University of Chicago Press.

Anitha, S. (2010). No recourse, no support: State policy and practice towards South Asian women facing domestic violence in the UK. *British Journal of Social Work*, 40(2), 462–479.

Australian Bureau of Statistics (ABS). (2014). *Average weekly earnings, Australia, May 2014*. Cat. No. 6302.0. Canberra, ACT: ABS.

Bacchi, C. (2009). *Analysing policy: what's the problem represented to be?* Sydney: Pearson.

Bak, C.K. and Larsen, J.E. (2015). Social exclusion or poverty individualisation? An empirical test of two recent and competing poverty theories. *European Journal of Social Work*, 18(1), 17–35.

Baker, C., Cook, S. and Norris, F. (2003). Domestic violence and housing problems: A contextual analysis of women's help-seeking, received informal support, and formal system response. *Violence Against Women*, 9(7), 754–783.

Baker, C.K., Niolon, P.H. and Oliphant, H. (2009). A descriptive analysis of transitional housing programs for survivors of intimate partner violence in the United States. *Violence Against Women*, 15(4), 460–481.

Baker, C., Billhardt, K., Warren, J., Rollins, C. and Glass, N. (2010). Domestic violence, housing instability, and homelessness: A review of housing policies and program practices for meeting the needs of survivors. *Aggression and Violent Behaviour*, 15(6), 430–439.

Baptista, I. (2010). Women and homelessness. (pp. 163–187). In E. O'Sullivan, V. Busch-Geertsema, D. Quilgars and N. Pleace (Eds). *Homelessness research in Europe*. Brussels: European Observatory on Homelessness.

Begun, S. and Walls, N.E. (2015). Pedestal or gutter: Exploring ambivalent sexism's relationship with abortion attitudes. *Affilia: Journal of Women and Social Work*, 30(2), 200–215.

Benjaminsen, L. (2014). 'Mindshift' and social work methods in a large-scale Housing First programme in Denmark. (pp. 12–13). In *FEANTSA Magazine: Social work in services with homeless people in a changing European social and political context*. Brussels: European Federation of National Organisations Working with the Homeless (AISBL).

Bessant, J. (2003). Pregnancy in a Brotherhood bin: Housing and drug-treatment options for pregnant young women. *Australian Social Work*, 56(3): 234–246.

Best, S. (2007). Culture turn. In G. Ritzer (Ed.). *Blackwell encyclopedia of sociology*. DOI: 10.1111/b.9781405124331.2007.x. Accessed 27 May 2015. www.blackwellreference.com/public/tocnode?id=g9781405124331_chunk_g97814051243319_ss1-202.

Bezunartea-Barrio, P. (2014). Social workers: Challenges and contributions to Housing First support programmes. (pp. 14–15). In *FEANTSA Magazine: Social work in services with homeless people in a changing European social and political context*. Brussels: European Federation of National Organisations Working with the Homeless (AISBL).

Blasi, G.L. (1990). Social policy and social science research on homelessness. *Journal of Social Issues*, 46, 207–219.

Blau, J. (1992). *The visible poor. Homelessness in the United States*. New York, NY: Oxford University Press.

Boes, M. and van Wormer, K. (1997). Social work with homeless women in emergency rooms: A strengths-feminist perspective. *Affilia: Journal of Women and Social Work*, 12(4), 408–426.

Bowie, S. and Dopwell, D. (2013). Metastressors as barriers to self-sufficiency among TANF-reliant African American and Latina women. *Affilia: Journal of Women and Social Work*, 28(2), 177–193.

Bowpitt, G., Dwyer, P., Sundin, E. and Weinstein, M. (2014). Places of sanctuary for 'the undeserving'? Homeless people's day centres and the problem of conditionality. *British Journal of Social Work*, 44, 1251–1267.

Broussard, C.A., Joseph, A.L. and Thompson, M. (2012). Stressors and coping strategies used by single mothers living in poverty. *Affilia: Journal of Women and Social Work*, 27(2), 190–204.

Browne, A. and Bassuk, S. (1997). Intimate violence in the lives of homeless and poor housed women: Prevalence and patterns in an ethnically diverse sample. *American Journal of Orthopsychiatry*, 67(2), 261–278.

Burrows, R., Pleace, N. and Quilgars, D. (Eds). (1997). *Homelessness and social policy*. London: Routledge.

Carlen, P. (1996). *Jigsaw: A political criminology of youth homelessness*. Buckingham, UK: Open University Press.

Casey, R., Goudie, R. and Reeve, K. (2008). Homeless women in public spaces: Strategies of resistance. *Housing Studies*, 23(6), 899–916.

Chamberlain, C. and MacKenzie, D. (2006). Homeless careers: A framework for intervention. *Australian Social Work*, 59(2), 198–212.

Chamberlain, C., Johnson, G. and Robinson, C. (Eds). (2014). *Homelessness in Australia: An introduction*. Sydney: University of New South Wales Press.

Chanmugam, A. (2014). Social work expertise and domestic violence fatality review teams. *Social Work*, 59(1), 73–80.

Christensen, A. and Jensen, S. (2012). Doing intersectional analysis: Methodological implications for qualitative research. *Nordic Journal of Feminist and Gender Research*, 20(2), 109–125.

Christian, J. (2003). Introduction. Special Issue: Homelessness: Integrating international perspectives. *Journal of Community and Applied Social Psychology*, 13(2), 85–90.

Christiani, A., Hudson, A.L., Nyamathi, A., Mutere, M. and Sweat, J. (2008). Attitudes of homeless and drug-using youth regarding barriers and facilitators in delivery of quality and culturally sensitive health care. *Journal of Child and Adolescent Psychiatric Nursing*, 21(3), 154–163.

Chung, D., Kennedy, R., O'Brien, B. and Wendt, S. (2000). *Home safe home: The link between domestic and family violence and women's homelessness*. Canberra, ACT: Partnerships Against Domestic Violence.

Clapham, D. (2005). *The meaning of housing*. Bristol, UK: Policy Press.

Clough, A., Draughon, J.E., Njie-Carr, V., Rollins, C. and Glass, N. (2014). 'Having housing made everything else possible': Affordable, safe and stable housing for women survivors of violence. *Qualitative Social Work*, 13(5), 671–688.

Cochran, B.N., Stewart, A.J., Ginzler, J.A., and Cauce, A. (2002). Challenges faced by homeless sexual minorities: Comparison of gay, lesbian, bisexual, and transgender homeless adolescents with their heterosexual counterparts. *American Journal of Public Health*, 92(5), 773–777.

Connolly, D.R. (2000). *Homeless mothers: Face to face with women and poverty*. Minneapolis, MN: University of Minnesota Press.

Corliss, H.L., Goodenow, C.S., Nichols, L. and Austin, S. (2011). High burden of homelessness among sexual-minority adolescents: Findings from a representative Massachusetts high school sample. *American Journal of Public Health*, 101(9), 1683–1689.

Cowan, D. (1999). Reforming the homeless legislation. *Critical Social Policy*, 18, 435–464.

Crath, R. (2012). Belonging as a mode of interpretive in-between: Image, place and space in the video works of racialised and homeless youth. *British Journal of Social Work*, 42(1), 42–57.

Culhane, D.P. (2008). The cost of homelessness: A perspective from the United States. *European Journal of Homelessness*, 2(1), 97–114.

Culhane, D.P., Metraux, S. and Hadley, T. (2002). Public service reductions associated with placement of homeless persons with severe mental illness in supportive housing. *Housing Policy Debate*, 13(1), 107–163.

De Winter, M. and Noom, M. (2003). Someone who treats you as an ordinary human being … Homeless youth examine the quality of professional care. *The British Journal of Social Work*, 33(3), 325–337.

Dewey, S. and Germain, T. (2014). Social services fatigue in domestic violence service provision facilities. *Affilia: Journal of Women and Social Work*, 29(4), 389–403.

Doherty, J. (2001). Gendering homelessness. (pp. 9–20). In B. Edgar, and J. Doherty (Eds). *Women and homelessness in Europe: Pathways, services and experiences*. Bristol, UK: Policy Press.

Doherty, J., Edgar, B. and Meert, H. (2004). *Homelessness research in the European Union*. Brussels: European Observatory on Homelessness.

Fitzpatrick, S. and Christian, J. (2006). Comparing homelessness research in the US and Britain. *International Journal of Housing Policy*, 6(3), 313–333.

Fitzpatrick, S., Johnsen, S. and Bramley, G. (2012). Multiple exclusion homelessness amongst migrants in the UK. *European Journal of Homelessness*, 6(1), 31–57.

Fortier, A. (2003). Making home: Queer migrations and motions of attachment. (pp. 115–135). In S. Ahmed, C. Castaneda, A. Fortier and M. Sheller (Eds). *Uprootings/regroundings: Questions of home and migration*. Oxford, UK: Berg.

Gibson, M. (2004). Melancholy objects. *Mortality*, 9(4), 285–299.

Goodkind, S. (2005). Gender-specific services in the juvenile justice system: A critical examination. *Affilia: Journal of Women and Social Work*, 20(1), 52–70.

Grace, M. and Gill, P.R. (2014). Improving outcomes for unemployed and homeless young people: Findings of the YP4 clinical controlled trial of joined up case management. *Australian Social Work*, 67(3), 419–437.

Graham, M. and Schiele, J.H. (2010). Equality-of-oppressions and anti-discriminatory models in social work: Reflections from the USA and UK. *European Journal of Social Work*, 13(2), 231–244.

Gressgård, R. (2008). Mind the gap: Intersectionality, complexity and 'the event'. *Theory and Science*, 10, 1–16.

Harding, R. and Hamilton, P. (2009). Working girls: Abuse or choice in street-level sex work? A study of homeless women in Nottingham. *British Journal of Social Work*, 39, 1118–1137.

Harrison, M. (1999). Theorising homelessness and 'race'. (pp. 101–121). In P. Kennett and A. Marsh (Eds). *Homelessness: Exploring the new terrain*. Bristol, UK: Policy Press.

Higate, P. (1997). Soldiering on? Theorising homelessness amongst ex-servicemen. (pp. 109–122). In R. Burrows, N. Pleace and D. Quilgars (Eds). *Homelessness and Social Policy*. London: Routledge.

hooks, bell. (1990). Homeplace: A site of resistance. (pp. 382–390). In *Yearning: Race, Gender and Cultural Politics*. Boston, MA: South End Press.

Horsell, C. (2006). Homelessness and social exclusion: A Foucauldian perspective for social workers. *Australian Social Work*, 59(2), 213–225.

Horsell, C. (2013). Homelessness, social policy and difference. *Advances in Social Work and Welfare Education*, 15(2), 39–55.

Horsell, C. (2014). Care, identity, social policy and homelessness. The Australian Sociological Association (TASA) Conference, University of South Australia, 24–27 November, Adelaide.

Hulko, W. (2015). Operationalizing intersectionality in feminist social work research: Reflections and techniques from research with equity-seeking groups. (pp. 69–89). In S. Wahab, B. Anderson-Nathe and C. Gringeri (Eds). *Feminisms in social work research*. New York: NY: Routledge.

Hutson, S. and Clapham, D. (Eds). (1999). *Homelessness: Public policies and private troubles*. London: Cassell.

Hutson, S. and Liddiard, M. (1994). *Youth homelessness: The construction of a social issue*. Basingstoke, UK: Macmillan.

Ignatieff, M. (2001). *Human rights as politics and idolatry*. Princeton, NJ: Princeton University Press.

Jacobs, K., Kemeny, J. and Manzi, T. (1999). The struggle to define homelessness: A constructivist approach. In S. Hutson and D. Clapham (Eds). *Homelessness: Public policies and private troubles*. London: Cassell.

Jasinski, J.L., Wesely, J.K., Wright, J.D. and Mustaine, E. (2010). *Hard lives, mean streets: Violence in the lives of homeless women*. Lebanon, NH: Northeastern University Press.

Jencks, C. (1994). *The homeless*. Cambridge, MA: Harvard University Press.

Johnson, A.K. (1989). Female-headed homeless families: A comparative profile. *Affilia: Journal of Women and Social Work*, 4(4), 23–39.

Johnson, A.K. (1995). Homelessness. In *Encyclopedia of social work* (19th ed.) (pp. 1338–1346). Washington, DC: National Association of Social Workers Press.

Johnson, A.K and Cnaan, R.A. (1995). Social work practice with homeless persons: State of the art. *Research on Social Work Practice*, 5(3), 340–382.

Johnson, A.K. and Kreuger, L.W. (1989). Toward a better understanding of homeless women. *Social Work*, 34(6), 537–540.

Johnson, A.K. and Richards, R.N. (1995). Homeless women and feminist social work practice. (pp. 232–257). In N. Van Den Berg (Ed.). *Feminist practice in the 21st century*. Washington, DC: National Association of Social Workers Press.

Johnson, G. and Chamberlain, C. (2008). Homelessness and substance abuse: Which comes first? *Australian Social Work*, 61(4), 342–356.

Johnson, G., Gronda, H. and Coutts, S. (2008). *On the outside: Pathways in and out of homelessness*. Melbourne, Vic: Australian Scholarly Publishing.

Jones, M., Shier, M. and Graham, J. (2012). Intimate relationships as routes into and out of homelessness: Insights from a Canadian city. *Journal of Social Policy*, 41, 101–117.

Jones, S. (Ed.). (2013). *Mean streets: A report on the criminalisation of homelessness in Europe*. Belgium: European Federation of National Organisations Working with the Homeless (FEANTSA), Housing Rights Watch, European Federation of National Associations Working with the Homeless (AISBL).

Kennedy, A. (2008). Eugenics, 'degenerate girls', and social workers during the progressive era. *Affilia: Journal of Women and Social Work*, 23(1), 22–37.

Kennett, P. and Marsh, A. (1999). *Homelessness: Exploring the new terrain*. Bristol, UK: Policy Press.

Klee, H. and Reid, P. (1998). Drug use among the young homeless: coping through self-medication. *Health*, 2, 115–134.

Krumer-Nevo, M., Berkovitz-Romano, A. and Komem, M. (2015). The study of girls in social work: Major discourses and feminist ideas. *Journal of Social Work*, 15(4), 425–446.

Kuhn, A. (2007). Photography and cultural memory: A methodological exploration. *Visual Studies*, 22(3), 283–292.

Laing, L. and Humphreys, C. (2013). *Social work and domestic violence*. London: Sage.

Liebow, E. (1995). *Tell them who I am: The lives of homeless women*. New York, NY: Penguin Books.

Lipmann, B. (2009). Elderly homeless men and women: Aged care's forgotten people. *Australian Social Work*, 6(2), 272–286.

Lykke, N. (2010a). *Feminist studies: A guide to intersectional theory, methodology, and writing*. New York, NY: Routledge.

Lykke, N. (2010b). The timeliness of post-constructionism. *NORA: Nordic Journal of Feminist and Gender Research*, 18(2), 131–136.

McArthur, M., Zubrzycki, J., Rochester, A. and Thomson, L. (2006). 'Dad, where are we going to live now?' Exploring fathers' experiences of homelessness. *Australian Social Work*, 59(3), 288–300.

McCall, L. (2005). The complexity of intersectionality. *Signs: Journal of Women in Culture and Society*, 30(3), 1771–1800.

McDowell, L. (1999). *Gender, identity and place: Understanding feminist geographies.* Oxford, UK: Polity Press.

McLaughlin, T.C. (2011). Using common themes: Cost-effectiveness of permanent supported housing for people with mental illness. *Research on Social Work Practice*, 21(4), 404–411.

Maeseele, T., Roose, R., Bouverne-De Bie, M. and Roets, G. (2014). From vagrancy to homelessness: The value of a welfare approach to homelessness. *British Journal of Social Work*, 44(7), 1717–1734.

Manthorpe, J., Cornes, M., Halloran, S. and Joly, L. (2015). Multiple exclusion homelessness: The preventive role of social work. *British Journal of Social Work*, 45(2), 587–599.

Martin, R. (2014). Gender and homelessness. (pp. 100–117). In C. Chamberlain, G. Johnson and C. Robinson (Eds). *Homelessness in Australia: An Introduction.* Sydney: University of New South Wales Press.

May, V.M. (2015). *Pursuing intersectionality: Unsettling dominant imaginaries.* New York, NY: Routledge.

Moore, T., McArthur, M. and Noble-Carr, D. (2011). Lessons learned from children who have experienced homelessness: What services need to know. *Children and Society*, 25(2), 115–126.

Mostowska, M. (2014). 'We shouldn't but we do…': Framing the strategies for helping homeless EU migrants in Copenhagen and Dublin. *British Journal of Social Work*, 44(1), 18–34.

Murphy, Y., Hunt, V., Zajicek, A.M., Norris, A.N. and Hamilton, L. (2009). *Incorporating intersectionality in social work practice, research, policy, and education.* Washington, DC: National Association of Social Workers Press.

Murray, S. (2011). Violence against homeless women: Safety and social policy. *Australian Social Work*, 64(3), 346–361.

Nixon, J. and Humphreys, C. (2010). Marshalling the evidence: Using intersectionality in the domestic violence frame. *Social Politics*, 17(2), 137–158.

Norris, A.N., Zajicek, A. and Murphy-Erby, Y. (2010). Intersectional perspective and rural poverty research: Benefits, challenges and policy implications. *Journal of Poverty*, 14(1), 55–75.

Nyamathi, A., Galaif, E.R. and Leake, B. (1999). A comparison of homeless women and their intimate partners. *Journal of Community Psychology*, 27(4), 489–502.

O'Sullivan, E., Busch-Geertsema, V., Quilgars, D. and Pleace, N. (2010). *Homelessness research in Europe.* Brussels: European Observatory on Homelessness.

Padgett, D.K., Gulcur, L. and Tsemberis, S. (2006). Housing first services for people who are homeless with co-occurring serious mental illness and substance abuse. *Research on Social Work Practice*, 16(1), 74–83.

Parsell, C. (2011). Responding to people sleeping rough: Dilemmas and opportunities for social work. *Australian Social Work*, 64(3), 330–345.

Passaro, J. (1996. Reprint 2014). *The unequal homeless: Men on the streets, women in their place.* London: Routledge.

Paterson, S. (2010). 'Resistors', 'helpless victims' and 'willing participants': The construction of women's resistance in Canadian anti-violence policy. *Social Politics*, 17(2), 159–184.

Pavao, J., Alvarez, J., Baumrind, N., Induni, M. and Kimerling, R. (2007). Intimate partner violence and housing instability. *American Journal of Preventive Medicine*, 32(2), 143–146.

Pearce, D. (1978). The feminization of poverty: Women, work and welfare. *The Urban and Social Change Review*, 11(1 and 2), 28–36.

Peressini, T. (2009). Pathways into homelessness: Testing the heterogeneity hypothesis. (Chapter 8.2). In J.D. Hulchanski, P. Campsie, S. Chau, S. Hwang and E. Paradis (Eds). *Finding home: Policy options for addressing homelessness in Canada* (e-book). Toronto: Cities Centre, University of Toronto. www.homelesshub.ca/FindingHome.

Pilkey, B. (2013). Embodiment of mobile homemaking imaginaries. *Geographical Research*, 51(2), 159–165.

Pink, S. (2007). *Doing visual ethnography: Images, media and representation in research* (2nd ed.). London: Sage.

Pleace, N. (2000). The new consensus, the old consensus and the provision of services for people sleeping rough. *Housing Studies*, 15(4), 581–594.

Pleace, N. (2010). Immigration and homelessness. (pp. 143–162). In E. O'Sullivan, V. Busch-Geertsema, D. Quilgars and N. Pleace (Eds). *Homelessness research in Europe*. Brussels: European Observatory on Homelessness.

Pleace, N. and Quilgars, D. (2003). Led rather than leading? Research on homelessness in Britain. *Journal of Community and Applied Social Psychology*, 13, 187–196.

Postmus, J.L., McMahon, S., Silva-Martinez, E. and Warrener, C.D. (2014). Exploring the challenges faced by Latinas experiencing intimate partner violence. *Affilia: Journal of Women and Social Work*, 29(4), 462–477.

Quigley, J., Raphael, S. and Smolensky, E. (2001). *Homelessness in California*. Berkeley, CA: Berkeley Program on Housing and Urban Policy.

Rich, K. (2014). 'My body came between us': Accounts of partner-abused women with physical disabilities. *Affilia: Journal of Women and Social Work*, 29(4), 418–433.

Roche, S. (2015). The salvaging of identities among homeless men: Reflections for social work. *Australian Social Work*, 68(2), 228–243.

Rossi, P. (1989a). *Without shelter: Homelessness in the 1980s*. New York, NY: Priority Press.

Rossi, P. (1989b). *Down and out in America: The origins of homelessness*. Chicago, IL: University of Chicago Press.

Rowntree, M. (2014). Making sexuality visible in Australian social work education. *Social Work Education*, 33(3), 353–364.

Rowntree, M. and Zufferey, C. (2015). Need or right: Sexual expression and intimacy in aged care. *Journal of Aging Studies*, 35, 20–25.

Russell, B. (1991. Reprint 2002 by Routledge). *Silent sisters: A study of homeless women*. New York, NY: Hemisphere Publishing.

Sandberg, L. (2013). Backward, dumb, and violent hillbillies? Rural geographies and intersectional studies on intimate partner violence. *Affilia: Journal of Women and Social Work*, 28(4), 350–365.

Scott, S. (2007). *All our sisters: Stories of homeless women in Canada*. Peterborough, ON: Broadview Press.

Shinn, M. and Weitzman, B.C. (1990). Research on homelessness: An introduction. *Journal of Social Issues*, 46, 1–11.

Shinn, M. and Weitzman, B.C. (1996). Homeless families are different. (pp. 109–122). In J. Baumohl (Ed.). *Homelessness in America*. Phoenix, AZ: Oryx Press.

Snow, D.A. and Anderson, L. (1987). Identity work among the homeless: The verbal construction and avowal of personal identities. *American Journal of Sociology*, 92, 1336–1371.

Snow, D.A. and Anderson, L. (1993). *Down on their luck: A study of homeless street people*. Berkeley, CA: University of California Press.

Sokoloff, N. and Dupont, I. (2005). Domestic violence at the intersections of race, class and gender: Challenges and contributions to understanding violence against marginalized women in diverse communities. *Violence Against Women*, 11(1), 38–64.

Somerville, P. (1992). Homelessness and the meaning of home: Rooflessness or rootlessness? *International Journal of Urban and Regional Research*, 16(4), 529–539.

Stewart, G. and Steward, J. (1992). Social work with homeless families. *British Journal of Social Work*, 22(3), 271–289.

Szeintuch, S. (2015). Street work and outreach: A social work method? *British Journal of Social Work*, 45(6), 1923–1934.

Tomas, A. and Dittmar, H. (1995). The experience of homeless women: an exploration of housing histories and the meaning of home. *Housing Studies*, 10(4), 493–513.

Vervliet, M., Jan De Mol, J., Eric Broekaert, E. and Derluyn, I. (2014). 'That I live, that's because of her': Intersectionality as framework for unaccompanied refugee mothers. *British Journal of Social Work*, 44(7), 2023–2041.

Voth Schrag, R.J. (2015). Economic abuse and later material hardship: Is depression a mediator? *Affilia: Journal of Women and Social Work*, 30(3), 341–351.

Wardhaugh, J. (1999).The unaccommodated woman: Home, homelessness and identity. *Sociological Review*, 47(1), 91–110.

Wasserman, J. and Clair, J. (2010). *At home on the street: People, poverty, and a hidden culture of homelessness*. Boulder, CO: Lynne Rienner.

Watkins, D.C., Hawkins, J. and Mitchell, J. (2015). The discipline's escalating whisper: Social work and black men's mental health. *Research on Social Work Practice*, 25(2), 240–250.

Watson, J. (2011). Understanding survival sex: Young women, homelessness and intimate relationships. *Journal of Youth Studies*, 14(6), 639–655.

Watson, S. (2000). Homelessness revisited: New reflections on old paradigms. *Urban Policy and Research*, 18(2), 159–170.

Watson, S. and Austerberry, H. (1986). *Housing and homelessness: A feminist perspective*. London: Routledge.

Williams, C. (1998). Domestic violence and poverty: The narratives of homeless women. *Frontiers*, 19(2), 143–160.

Williams, C. (2003). *'A roof over my head': Homeless women and the shelter industry*. Boulder, CO: University Press of Colorado.

Williams, M. and Cheal, B. (2001). Is there any such thing as homelessness? Measurement, explanation and process in 'homelessness' research. *Innovation: The European Journal of Social Science Research*, 14(3), 239–253.

Wright, J.D. (1988). *The worthy and unworthy homeless. Society*, 25, 64–69.

Wright, J. and Rubin, B. (1991). Is homelessness a housing problem? *Housing Policy Debate*, 2(3), 937–956.

Wright, T. (1997). *Out of place: Homeless mobilizations, subcities, and the contested landscape*. Albany, NY: State University of New York Press.

Yamada, A.M., Werkmeister Rozas, L.M. and Cross-Denny, B. (2015). Intersectionality and social work. In *Encyclopaedia of social work*. Washington, DC: NASW and Oxford University Press. DOI: http://dx.doi.org/10.1093/acrefore/9780199975839.013.961.

Yuval-Davis, N. (2006). Intersectionality and feminist politics. *European Journal of Women's Studies*, 13(3), 193–209.

Yuval-Davis, N. (2011). *The politics of belonging*. London: Sage.

Zufferey, C. (2008). Responses to homelessness in Australian cities: Social worker perspectives. *Australian Social Work*, 61(4), 357–371.

Zufferey, C. (2009a). Making gender visible: Social work responses to homelessness. *Affilia: Journal of Women and Social Work*, 24(4), 382–393.

Zufferey, C. (2009b). Teaching about homelessness with a focus on children and families, as an emerging area of social work practice. *Advances in Social Work and Welfare Education*, 11(1), 109–116.

Zufferey, C. (2015). Diverse meanings of home in multicultural Australia. *The International Journal of Diverse Identities*, 13(2), 13–21.

Zufferey, C. (2016). Homelessness and intersectional feminist practice. (pp. 238–249). In S. Wendt and N. Moulding (Eds). *Contemporary feminisms in social work practice*. Abingdon, UK: Routledge.

Zufferey, C. and Chung, D. (2015). 'Red dust homelessness': housing, home and homelessness in remote Australia. *Journal of Rural Studies*, 41, 13–22.

Zufferey, C. and Kerr, L. (2004). Identity and everyday experiences of homelessness: Some implications for social work. *Australian Social Work*, 57(4), 343–353.

Zufferey, C. and Rowntree, M. (2014). Finding your community wherever you go? Exploring how a group of women who identify as lesbian embody and imagine 'home'. The Australian Sociological Association (TASA) Conference, University of South Australia, 24–27 November, Adelaide.

Zufferey, C., Chung, D., Franzway, S., Wendt, S. and Moulding, N. (2016). Intimate partner violence and housing: Eroding women's citizenship. *Affilia: Journal of Women and Social Work*. DOI: 10.1177/0886109915626211.

4 Social policy and homelessness

This chapter discusses multidisciplinary literature that examines the incorporation of intersectionality in policy development and analysis. I explore different policy-making and analysis approaches, focusing on Olena Hankivsky's (2012b) Intersectionality-Based Policy Analysis (IBPA) and Carol Bacchi's (2009) 'What's the problem represented to be?'(WPR). I critically examine definitions of homelessness in the USA, UK, Australia, the EU and New Zealand, and the widespread implementation of homelessness programmes such as Housing First. I also discuss Parken's (2010) multi-strand approach that provides a step forward in institutionalising intersectional theorising in policy making. In this chapter I argue that policy research grounded in intersectionality can contribute to improving policy approaches to homelessness, especially by highlighting unequal power relations in the policy-making process.

Background

Intersectionality has been used as a theoretical policy inquiry by scholars in the legal field (commencing with Kimberlee Crenshaw), in gender and politics (Yuval-Davis, 2006; Lombardo and Verloo, 2009), in public policy (such as Wilkinson, 2003), in sociology (Strid *et al.*, 2013) and in health policy (Hankivsky, 2012a). In relation to social policy and social work, Murphy *et al.* (2009) and Bowie and Dopwell (2013) discuss the importance of intersectionality. Public policy and political science scholar Tiffany Manuel (2006, pp. 194–195) argues that because public policy is 'reductionist' and 'incremental', there are many challenges involved in incorporating intersectionality into traditional research and policy paradigms. The concern is that policy-making processes will simplify intersecting experiences of privilege and oppression (Wilkinson, 2003). There is a dearth of theorising about homelessness social policy making using intersectionality in social work literature. Therefore, this chapter draws on multidisciplinary intersectional policy analysis to examine definitions of homelessness and Housing First responses to the issue.

As previously mentioned, when first coined by Crenshaw, intersectionality was used as a tool to analyse discrimination legislation, in order to make visible the effects of policy making on African American women. Therefore, from its origins, intersectional policy analysis highlighted intersecting structural oppressions that marginalised particular population groups (Manuel, 2006). McCall's (2005) categorical approaches can also contribute to intersectional policy analysis because policy making and analysis can be influenced by inter-categorical, intra-categorical and anti-categorical approaches. Using inter-categorical research and policy tools, inequalities between fixed and preselected groups can be measured across multiple dimensions, including how categories and inequalities change over time, such as wage indicators and income differences (McCall, 2005, p. 1790). The intra-categorical policy analysis approach can assist researchers to examine diversity within disadvantaged (and privileged) population groups (McCall, 2005). This can be seen in Asmara Carbado's (2012) MA in Afro-American Studies, which employs the theory of intersectionality. Her thesis examines the 1806 Virginia Supreme Court decision, Hudgins v. Wright and how race is intersectionally constituted in legal processes. She argues that intra-categorical intersectionality is useful for examining the process by which a number of factors, such as physical appearance, gender, family background, white witnesses, reputation and judges' personal views on slavery intersect to construct race in court processes (Carbado, 2012). As well, in the UK context, when theorising racism, social work scholar Masocha (2015) has focused on xenoracism (nationalism and racism). He examined racism in media representations and policy responses to asylum seekers, highlighted social work perspectives that counter hegemonic narratives about asylum seekers, as well as perspectives that engage in exclusionary processes that construct the Other (such as asylum seekers). As discussed in the previous chapter, I have drawn on an anti-categorical approach to deconstruct and unsettle dominant policy assumptions about homelessness as 'houselessness' (Zufferey and Chung, 2015), which will be further expanded on in this chapter. The social justice values that underpin intersectional policy analysis and research resonate with the ethics of social work. However, little social work research on intersectionality, homelessness and social policy could be found in literature.

Social work authors Norris *et al.* (2010, p. 63) note that policy-oriented scholars do articulate intersectional concepts. Building on Crenshaw's (1991) ideas about over-inclusion and under-inclusion, they argue, however, that scholars have tended to emphasise one inequality analytically over intersecting multiple inequalities (Norris *et al.*, 2010). Over-inclusion and under-inclusion can occur, when for example, theorising race and gender (Norris *et al.*, 2010, p. 63; May, 2015). For example, when policy makers assume that 'Black women's political and economic interests will be achieved by meeting the demand for racial equality', gender inequalities in Black communities are silenced and thus the 'interests of Black men' are privileged (Norris, *et al.*, 2010, p. 63). Both gendered and racialised social inequalities intersect and constitute experiences of homelessness, along with other aspects, such as sexual orientation, disability, age, class, geographical location, religion and experiences of migration, being a refugee and experiencing violence. Therefore, intersectional policy making and analysis can explore how policies respond to intersecting and multiple discriminations simultaneously.

Incorporating intersectionality in policy making and analysis

Intersectionality has been used by social work scholars to develop, assess, evaluate, analyse and advocate for social research and policies that incorporate at least two or more 'categories of oppression' (Hulko, 2015, p. 71). This is relevant when examining policy responses to homelessness and considering if social policies are inclusive of intersecting diversities (Zufferey, 2015). However, intersectionality literature has tended to focus on 'theoretical disagreement and abstract debates' (Strid *et al.*, 2013, p. 559). Few authors have explored how intersectionality is institutionalised in policy practice or social architecture (Verloo *et al.*, 2012). Authors such as Lombardo and Verloo (2009) in Europe, Strid *et al.* (2013) in the UK and Bowie and Dopwell (2013) in the USA are notable for drawing on intersectionality to examine policies and policy-making processes.

In Europe, Verloo (2006) from the Netherlands, and Lombardo (Lombardo and Verloo, 2009) from Spain, examined reforms to equality law in European Union (EU) member states that aimed to address discrimination about gender, race and ethnicity, religion and belief, age, disability and sexuality. Lombardo and Verloo (2009, p. 479) contend that Crenshaw's concept of 'political intersectionality' can enable 'policymakers and activists to reflect on the dynamics of privilege and exclusion that emerge when people at the intersections of different inequalities are overlooked'. However, despite the Charter of Fundamental Rights of the European Union (2000), Verloo (2006) and Lombardo and Verloo (2009) argue that the EU response to the equality agenda from the Amsterdam Treaty onwards has been contested. This was evident when two separate but similar institutions – the European Institute for Gender Equality and the Fundamental Rights Agency – were created, reflecting alliances and contestations within European civil society (Lombardo and Verloo, 2009). Verloo (2006) highlighted few examples of intersectional responses and policies found in the United Nations that intersected race and gender. For example, in 2004, the 'Committee on the Elimination of Racial Discrimination adopted a general recommendation on gender-related dimensions of racial discrimination (CRD/56/Misc21/Rev.3)'. As well, in 2001, The Commission on the Status of Women organised a panel on 'Gender and all forms of discrimination, in particular racism, racial discrimination, xenophobia and related intolerance' at its 45th session (Verloo, 2006, p. 214). More recently, Rashida Manjoo, Special Rapporteur on Violence Against Women for the United Nations (UN) Human Rights Council (United Nations General Assembly, 2014) argued that the intersectionality of political, economic, social, cultural, and gender factors obscure and exacerbate violence against women across the world, which also potentially shapes women's experiences of homelessness.

The equity policies of the EU have traditionally tackled each equity strand (gender, race and ethnicity, disability, sexual orientation and nationality) separately, such as through the introduction of the Racial Equality Directive, Employment Equality Directive 2000 and Equal Treatment Directive 2002, each covering different forms of discrimination (Kantola, 2009). In a move towards addressing equality mainstreaming and multiple discriminations, the focus has shifted away from gender and towards racial discrimination, which has 'created unrest amongst feminists in European politics and law' (Kantola, 2009, p. 22). Verloo (2006, p. 211) noted that policy practice 'seldom refers to intersectionality when trying to deal with multiple inequalities' and that intersections are rarely addressed in EU policies. She argued that 'one size fits all' policy approaches addressing multiple discriminations are based on an incorrect assumption of sameness and ignores the processes that constitute inequalities (Verloo, 2006, p. 211). Lombardo and Verloo (2009, p. 478) conclude that the EU legal framework is 'juxtaposing inequalities rather than intersecting them and is not giving equal importance to the different inequalities'. Therefore, as inequalities are framed and experienced differently, the challenge for policy makers would be to respond to intersecting social inequalities, as well as differences and similarities between and within different population groups.

Similarly, Kantola and Nousiainen (2009, p. 459) from Finland and Turkey, draw a distinction between 'intersectionality' and 'multiple discrimination' and argued that 'the EU focuses on the latter ... favouring anti-discrimination policy'. Whilst these policies are intended to tackle multiple and intersecting discriminations, political and legal institutions such as marriage, parenting and inheritance law govern and reproduce inequalities and have the power to remedy some inequalities and 'ignore and silence others' (Kantola and Nousiainen, 2009, p. 462). They note that inequalities can differ according to 'choice' (for example, a person can choose his/her religion but not their age) and 'visibility' (for example, sexuality can be hidden but gender or skin colour cannot), and that social locations can change over time (for example, age and disability alter over time but most people will not change their sex). These social markers are then responded to in various ways in different social institutions (Kantola and Nousiainen, 2009, p. 468) that can be oppressive or privileging.

In the UK, Strid et al. (2013) emphasised that intersectionality is particularly important for policy making. They analysed British policies (2001–2011) on domestic violence (which included homelessness), sexual violence and forced marriage, to show how intersectionality can improve policy. When examining multiple inequalities, such as 'age, class, disability, ethnicity/race, gender, immigrant status, religion/belief and sexual orientation', they argued that there are different (but limited) visibilities of multiple inequalities

(Strid *et al.*, 2013, p. 566). They identified the following three different vis-ibilities: when inequalities are simply named in policies (which is the least inclusive and visible), when 'intersecting inequalities, fields and domains' are highlighted in policies and when 'the voices of minoritised women' are included in the policy process, with 'outcomes through civil society', such as the development of coalitions and alliances between women's organisa-tions (Strid *et al.*, 2013, pp. 566, 599). A number of authors have claimed that multiple inequalities and intersectionality are invisible in policies on vio-lence against women (Nixon and Humphreys, 2010; Hankivsky and Cormier, 2011; Zufferey *et al.*, 2016). On the other hand, Strid *et al.*'s (2013, p. 574) analysis of British policies on sexual assault, domestic violence and forced marriages note that the inclusion of intersecting inequalities in policies range from 'weak inclusion in policy on sexual offences' (that is, simply the naming of differences), to 'moderate inclusion in policy on domestic violence' and strong inclusion of minoritised women's voices in shaping 'policy on forced marriage' (Strid *et al.*, 2013, p. 574) consistent with the social justice aims of intersectionality. However, these authors also noted that domestic violence policies and legislation are increasingly degendered, and whilst degendered aspects can be intersectional, 'violence against women cannot be efficiently combated when policy is degendered to the point where gender becomes invis-ible' (Strid *et al.*, 2013, p. 575). This would be equally relevant to intersecting gender with other categories of disadvantage in homelessness policies, includ-ing focusing specifically on both women's and men's homelessness. However, when examining Australian homelessness policy, I found that discussions of power and gender inequalities are often missing (Zufferey, 2011).

In the US policy context, Bowie and Dopwell (2013, p. 190) argued that intersectionality research is a viable alternative when examining the outcomes and the flaws of the Temporary Assistance for Needy Families (TANF) programme. These flaws include its contradictory logic about employment searches, work incentives and the lack of available living-wage jobs. They argued that intersectional research of the TANF programme can highlight social and policy inequalities, such as:

(1) the social and political construction of TANF; (2) its emphasis on mac-roinstitutional and microintimate partner power relations (e.g., TANF-reliant women, public welfare case managers, and low-wage employers in the business community) that create and sustain social hierarchies; and (3) the perspectives and experiences of different oppressed groups, espe-cially women of color, and (4) it is interdisciplinary and driven by the pursuit of social justice.

(Bowie and Dopwell, 2013, p. 190)

The policy-making process involves an assessment of social justice, society's wellbeing and the distribution of finite resources to address it (Murphy *et al.*, 2009, p. 62). According to Bowie and Dopwell (2013, pp. 177–178),

President Franklin Delano Roosevelt's New Deal that responded to the economic crisis of the early 1930s was an early example of this process, resulting in 'the creation of what was perceived to be a socially just minimum safety net for low-income and impoverished Americans'. As a component of the Social Security Act of 1935, the federal government created Aid to Dependent Children (which later became Aid to Families with Dependent Children, AFDC) and provided cash assistance to eligible poor families. The Personal Responsibility and Work Opportunity Reconciliation Act of 1996 (PRWORA) abolished AFDC and replaced it with Temporary Assistance for Needy Families (TANF). The TANF is an income support programme with a 'work first philosophy' and 'strict enforcement of welfare-to-work guidelines, penalties and financial sanctions for noncompliance with regulations and more restrictive eligibility criteria' (Bowie and Dopwell, 2013, pp. 177–178). These policies are particularly relevant to families who are homeless and poor in the USA.

Bowie and Dopwell's (2013) study focused on the 'metastressors', such as labour market issues, housing and environmental issues, family stressors, interpersonal violence, mental and physical ill-health and barriers to employment and career outcomes, as experienced by 30 TANF-reliant African and Latino women. They argued that TANF structures and regulations are designed to 'control and oppress women, particularly those who are single, impoverished and heads of households', and that by design, the public welfare system 'perpetuates poverty, second-class citizenship and inequality in the United States' (Bowie and Dopwell, 2013, p. 179). These policies purposely 'contribute to providing low wage labor' while state-defined 'success' means exiting from TANF assistance, which can then exacerbate family, community and social problems (Bowie and Dopwell, 2013, p. 179). For example, many people living in poverty are employed but their wages are too low to pay for housing. This state of affairs reflects the residual approach to social welfare in the United States, the United Kingdom and Australian welfare systems (Esping-Andersen, 1990). Whilst welfare policies and service responses are intended to ameliorate disadvantage, structural or institutional inequalities can be ignored, including persistent homophobia, racism or sexism faced by diverse population groups when accessing employment or housing.

Intersectionality is useful to highlight the intersecting complexities that constitute social policy-making processes, and to examine whose voices are heard and whose voices are missing in policy development (Bowie and Dopwell, 2013). Whilst academic scholars are committed to addressing inequalities through intersectionality, as an instrument of political and social change, social policies have been critiqued for failing to address 'experiences of intersectional discrimination', especially for marginalised women (Ferree, 2009; Norris *et al.*, 2010, p. 63). Social policies (such as those addressing homelessness) can risk privileging some and ignoring other social inequalities, reproducing power relations and failing to address intersecting inequalities that constitute homelessness. It remains important to ask who defines the differences (and similarities) that are recognised in policy making and 'when, where, which and why' are these of focus (Ludvig, 2006, p. 247). These relations of power are important to consider when examining social policy responses to homelessness, such as how intersections are presented, in relation to competing categorisations of social inequalities. To incorporate intersectionality and address intersecting power differentials, policy-making and policy analysis becomes complicated.

Policy analysis approaches

There are different models about the cyclic stages in policy making. These models range from simpler four stage models involving planning, formulation, implementation and evaluation, to more complicated eight stage ones, that include issue identification, policy analysis, policy instrumentation, consultation, coordination, decision making, implementation and evaluation (Carson and Kerr, 2014, p. 85). Social work policy makers rely on multidisciplinary assessments and assume that many different interests and government entities are involved in a multi-staged and continuous policy process (Murphy *et al.*, 2009, pp. 59–60). Drawing on Dunn's (1994) public policy model of analysis, Murphy *et al.* (2009) argue that policy definition, agenda setting, policy adoption, policy implementation and policy evaluation are relevant to social work practice. They call for social workers to be involved in all stages of the policy-making process as well as policy research, analysis, advocacy and critique.

Policy making and analysis is varied and contested. Mayer *et al.* (2004, p. 15) argue that there are six different styles of policy analysis, which asks different questions. For example, the rational style asks 'What is good knowledge?'; the argumentative style asks 'What is good for the debate?'; the client advice style asks 'What is good for the client/problem owner?'; the participatory style asks 'What is good for democratic society?'; the process style asks 'What is good for the process?'; and the interactive style asks 'What is good for mutual understanding?' Murphy *et al.* (2009, p. 60) note that social workers utilise an eclectic approach to policy analysis that incorporates aspects of these different policy theories. Social work policy analysis in the field of homelessness can include any (or a mix of) these styles, depending on the purposes of the analysis.

In Canada, intersectionality has been used to assist health care scholars and policy analysts to question 'how is policy done?' (Hankivsky and Cormier, 2011, p. 220). Hankivsky and her colleagues (Hankivsky and Christoffersen, 2008; Hankivsky and Cormier, 2009; Hankivsky and Cormier, 2011; Hankivsky, 2011; Hankivsky, 2012a; 2012b; Hankivsky *et al.*, 2014) have developed Intersectionality-Based Policy Analysis (IBPA) as a framework for analysing health and public policy. Hankivsky and Cormier (2011) discuss different theoretical approaches to intersectional public policy analysis. One potential approach replaces the notion of 'context' with 'space' as an analytical dimension in intersectionality policy analysis. This theoretical shift includes historically contextualising policies, the purposes and authors of the text, how power dimensions are re-produced in the text and the relationships between power and agency (Rönnblom, 2008, p. 2). This approach to intersectional policy analysis is potentially relevant to examining exclusionary policy responses to homelessness in urban places and spaces (Zufferey, 2016). Urban space scholars refer to 'new geographies' of wealth and exclusion, 'shelter deprivation' and cities being constituted by unequal social, economic and political relations, with class, race, ethnicity and gender continuing to be 'key markers of urban inequality' (Stevenson, 2013, p. 3; Tonkiss, 2013, p. 22). As Kennelly and Watt (2011, p. 768) argue, 'urban spaces are not neutral … they carry the weight of political, social and cultural processes that create distinctive areas of leisure, employment, housing and destitution'. Thus, urban policy responses potentially increase the polarisation between the rich and poor and the surveillance of more marginalised population groups, such as people who experience literal homelessness.

An intersectional policy analysis approach can also focus on reconceptualising policy initiatives at different stages of the policy cycle, through using case studies. For example, Murphy *et al.* (2009, p. 67) applied intersectional policy process analysis to a case study (Natalia) about sex trafficking. In their intersectional policy analysis they include: exploring the social, political and economic definition of the problem; determining who is central to the agenda setting and adoption of the policy; identifying what agencies will implement the policy; and determining how the policy can be evaluated (Murphy *et al.*, 2009). As well, Bishwakarma *et al.* (2007 p. 34) examined Nepalese education policy strategies developed within the Tenth Development Plan (2002–2007) and their 'effectiveness' in addressing the exclusion of Dalit (oppressed or 'untouchable') women, through 'the lens of the intersection of caste and gender'. These authors strived to systematically integrate intersectionality in the policy-making and analysis processes. Whilst these authors are not all social workers, I posit that intersectional policy analysis can also be used effectively by social workers who make and analyse policy in the field of homelessness.

In this chapter, I ask intersectional policy analysis questions to examine statutory policy definitions of homelessness that can shape social work practice in the USA, UK, Australia and the European Union. As well, I examine Housing First policy responses to homelessness in the USA, UK, Canada, Europe and Australia. First, I will outline the questions posed in two policy analysis frameworks: Hankivsky's (2012b) IBPA and Bacchi's (2009) 'What's the problem represented to be?' (WPR). These frameworks are used to question homelessness policy definitions in the USA, UK, Australia and the EU, and to examine the implementation of Housing First initiatives.

Policy analysis frameworks: Intersectionality-Based Policy Analysis (IBPA) and 'What's the problem represented to be?' (WPR)

The notion of Intersectionality-Based Policy Analysis (IBPA) provides a new method for understanding equity based implications of policy. This approach aims to promote improvements in policy development and highlight social justice for diverse population groups, especially in health policy (Hankivsky, 2012a; 2012b). IBPA offers guiding principles for examining intersecting categories, which includes reflecting on multilevel analyses of power, reflexivity, time and space, giving voice to diverse knowledges, as well as advocating for social justice and equity. Hankivsky *et al.* (2014, p. 1) argue that IBPA is a critical policy analysis that 'captures the different dimensions of policy contexts, including history, politics, everyday lived experiences, diverse knowledges and intersecting social locations', and that 'generates transformative insights' and policy solutions. However, IBPA has predominantly been used in public and health policies, and I have not been able to find its application to any homelessness policy development or analysis in social work literature.

Intersectionality-Based Policy Analysis (IBPA)[1] consists of five descriptive questions and seven transformative questions. The five *descriptive* questions start with self-reflexivity, examining historical constructions of contemporary problems (such as homelessness) and outlining policy intentions. These questions ask: What knowledge, values and experiences do you bring to this area of policy analysis? What is the policy 'problem' under consideration? How have representations of the 'problem' come about? How are groups differentially affected by this representation of the 'problem'? What are the current policy responses trying to achieve? (Hankivsky, 2012b, pp. 39–40). The seven Intersectionality-Based Policy Analysis (IBPA) *transformative* questions ask: What inequities actually exist in relation to the problem and what potential approaches can be used to promote discussion of the problem? Where and how can interventions be made to improve the problem? What are feasible short-, medium- and long-term solutions? How will proposed policy responses reduce inequities and promote social justice? How will implementation and uptake be assured? How will you know if inequities have been reduced? How has the process of engaging in an intersectionality-based policy analysis transformed thinking about relations and structures of power and inequity? (Hankivsky, 2012b, pp. 40–42). One example of an intersectional policy process is Parken's (2010) Multi-Strand Method in the UK, which is discussed later in the chapter. As well, service user-led research in Housing First by 'The People with Lived Experience Caucus' in Canada (Coltman *et al.*, 2015) is also an example of inclusive intersectional research and policy practice, which is mentioned in this chapter, but further discussed in Chapter 6. Potentially both examples are innovative approaches to intersectional policy implementation and evaluation, incorporating intersecting inequalities and the diverse voices of service users.

The five IBPA descriptive questions are similar to Bacchi's (2009, p. vii) 'What's the problem represented to be?' (WPR) framework that deconstructs the 'problem solving' discourse in public policy, through a 'problem questioning' policy analysis. The WPR approach provides an analysis of the policy process of 'governing' (such as by social workers), in relation to people who are 'governed' (Bacchi, 2009, p. vii), such as people who are defined as homeless. The WPR methodology includes the following questions: What is the problem represented to be in a specific policy? What presuppositions or assumptions underlie this representation of the problem? How has this representation of the problem come about? What is left unproblematic in this problem representation? Where are the silences? Can the problem be thought about differently? What effects are produced by this representation of the problem? How/where has this representation of the problem been produced, disseminated and defended? How could it be questioned, disrupted and replaced? (Bacchi, 2009, p. 2). This WPR policy analysis framework, which is more post structural in emphasis, resonates with the anti-categorical approach (McCall, 2005) that can assist social workers to deconstruct the problematising of homelessness in policy responses.

When examining the effects of policy discourses on individual subjectivities, Bacchi (2009, p. 15) identifies three interconnecting effects of particular representations of social problems such as homelessness. The first are discursive effects (for example, the limits that are imposed on what can be thought of and said about homelessness). The second are subjectification effects (for example, how the subjectivities of people experiencing homelessness are constituted in media and policy discourse). The third are lived experience effects, for example, the impact of these representations on the experiences of people subjected to the discourse/s of homelessness (Zufferey, 2014). I have previously utilised the WPR approach to examine print media representations of homelessness in Australia and found that public depictions of people who experience homelessness can reinforce deep-seated community values that maintain unequal gender, class and racialised power relations. These social constructions, such as expecting social workers to 'fix' problems such as homelessness, frequently ignore the strengths and agency of service users (Zufferey, 2014, p. 527).

Intersectional policy analysis requires an understanding and assessment of how power is produced and unevenly distributed through society's social structures, institutions, organisations and 'everyday interactions' (Murphy *et al.*, 2009, p. 62). The examination of 'interlocking structures of oppression' is valuable for analysing social inequalities and the impact of policies on different social groups (Murphy *et al.*, 2009, p. 62), including people who experience homelessness. When considering relevant policies, it is important to highlight statutory definitions of homelessness that are designed primarily to ration access to public resources, within particular welfare state contexts and unequal power relations.

Problem definition and agenda setting in homelessness

Problem definition in policy making is a 'matter of representation', which is connected to how a social problem (such as homelessness) is constructed and promoted by strategic lobby groups (Murphy *et al.*, 2009, p. 61). In the agenda-setting phase, policy makers negotiate social issues for government action, as influenced by political lobbying and diverse community groups (Murphy *et al.*, 2009, p. 60; Carson and Kerr, 2014). Homelessness has historically been responded to by the voluntary sector and non-government agencies, as powerful lobby groups in this field of practice.

Alongside lobby groups (such as non-government agencies), the news media can shape policy agendas and contribute to increasing public awareness and concern for salient issues such as homelessness. The news media does not only reflect reality but filters and shapes it. The media interest on particular issues such as homelessness can influence the public to perceive that some social issues are more important than others, and can homogenise and promote standardised definitions and solutions to the issue (Zufferey, 2014). Reflecting media representations of homelessness, policy responses to homelessness have concentrated on literal, primary or visible homelessness, such as 'rough sleeping' in Britain and Australia, and 'street people' in America, or housing chronically homeless people who are deemed to be costly to the government (Stanhope and Dunn, 2011). These 'chronically homeless' are currently being responded to through Housing First policies and service initiatives. However, attention on homelessness as 'rough sleeping' and on chronic homelessness means that policies have tended to concentrate on men, who are more likely to experience and remain literally and chronically homeless (Passaro, 1996/2014). The next section examines how homelessness is statutorily defined in the USA, UK, Australia, European Union and New Zealand. It asks questions about how policies and legislation represent and respond to homelessness and what is missing when thinking about policies using intersectional policy analysis.

Statutory definitions of homelessness

In the USA, the Stewart B. McKinney Homeless Act of 1987 (Pub L. No.100–77) was the first federal law that provided money for emergency food and homeless shelters. In 2009, President Obama signed the Homeless Emergency Assistance and Rapid Transition to Housing (HEARTH) Act of 2009, which now emphasises permanent supportive housing and rapid re-housing (within 30 days). This strategy is consistent with the Housing First approaches also being promoted in Europe, the UK and Australia. In addition, Section 103 of the McKinney-Vento Homeless Assistance Act (42 U.S.C. 11302) has amended statutory definitions in Sec. 1003 of the HEARTH Act, which covers an individual or family who lacks an 'adequate night time residence', such as living in a car, park, abandoned building, bus or train station, airport, camping ground or 'place not meant for human habitation', living in a service/ shelter, as well as people 'at risk' of imminently losing housing, including those that people own, rent or live in. This Act also legislates to respond to chronicity and 'life threatening conditions', which highlights multiple social inequalities:

> chronic disabilities, chronic physical health or mental health conditions, substance addiction, histories of domestic violence or childhood abuse, the presence of a child or youth with a disability, or multiple barriers to employment [as well as] any individual or family who is fleeing, or is attempting to flee, domestic violence, dating violence, sexual assault, stalking, or other dangerous or life-threatening conditions [and] lack the resources or support networks to obtain other permanent housing.
>
> (HEARTH Act, 2009, Sec. 1003)

This definition concentrates on chronic homelessness but also represents the issue as covering people 'at risk' of losing their housing and experiencing domestic violence. Thus, this definition moves beyond the category of homelessness being 'street people'. As such, homelessness is represented as being related to chronic health conditions, disabilities and addictions, as well as emergencies and access to resources. The policy does cover multiple social issues but does not consider how they intersect, how unequal power relations are produced and how discriminatory practices contribute to homelessness. For example, persistent and institutionalised racialised, gendered and classed discrimination in housing, employment and health policies and practices particularly affect African American individuals, families and communities, who are more likely to become homeless and have lower homeownership rates (Jewell, 2003).

In Britain, the original (as enacted) Housing (Homeless Persons Act) 1977 Section 1 defined homelessness as lack of housing: 'no accommoda- tion, or accommodation which he/she cannot secure entry to'. Furthermore, homelessness includes if one's housing is a 'movable structure, vehicle or ves- sel designed or adapted for human habitation ... with no place where he is entitled or permitted both to place it and to reside in it'. Thus, the original UK definition of homelessness covers people 'sleeping rough' (such as on the streets or in a car or 'moveable structure'); those staying in temporary homeless accommodation and also those about to lose their accommodation ('threatened with homelessness'), or living in 'unreasonable' accommoda- tion, where it is substandard or there is a threat of domestic violence (Robson and Poustie, 1996). The specific reference to 'domestic' violence was edited in 2002, now defined more broadly as: '(a) violence from another person; or (b) threats of violence from another person which are likely to be carried out' (Homelessness Act 2002, Section 10). The Acts also discussed local housing authorities developing homelessness strategies to prevent homelessness, secure sufficient accommodation and provide 'satisfactory provision of support for people in their district who are or may become homeless'. However, despite the rhetorical intent of these policies, they have not contributed to transforming power relations.

In tracing the history of the development of this Act, Crowson (2012, p. 23) argues that although faith-based lobby groups shaped and framed the public debate about homelessness from the late 1950s onwards, they have had 'little direct control over the creation and amendment of legislation'. Crowson (2012) noted that political institutions implementing government policies are constituted by heteronormative, racialised and classed discourses that continue to view homelessness as an individual, welfare issue. For example, people who are homeless continue to be constructed as victims and represented as 'marginal and troublesome' (Meers, 2012). Furthermore, this Act was critiqued for institutionalising the notion of 'intentional' and 'unintentional' homelessness, and responding to people only within locality-based connections (such as local government areas), which did not reduce transient homelessness and housing shortages (Crowson, 2012). Furthermore, according to section 186, 'an asylum-seeker, or a dependant of an asylum-seeker' is ineligible for housing assistance in the United Kingdom.

The original Housing (Homeless Persons) Act 1977, Section 2 also defined priority need for accommodation. The Housing Act 1996 and Homelessness Act 2002 defined priority need for accommodation in Section 189 as:

> (a) a pregnant woman or a person with whom she resides or might reasonably be expected to reside; (b) a person with whom dependent children reside or might reasonably be expected to reside; (c) a person who is vulnerable as a result of old age, mental illness or handicap or physical disability or other special reason, or with whom such a person resides or might reasonably be expected to reside; (d) a person who is homeless or threatened with homelessness as a result of an emergency such as flood, fire or other disaster.

This response to homelessness focuses on prioritising 'disadvantaged' population groups, on the basis of social need categories, such as pregnancy, children, age, ability, socioeconomic status and mental health. The provision of statutory homelessness assistance is reported to have improved for families with dependents (Fitzpatrick and Pleace, 2012, p. 246). However, single people without serious health issues have tended to be defined as less deserving and are more often, intentionally homeless (Fitzpatrick and Pleace, 2012, p. 246; Crowson, 2012). The term 'vulnerable' has also been critiqued for being too vague, acting as a 'gate keeping' device for local housing authorities in deciding who is 'vulnerable' and in practice, encouraging a deserving/underserving mentality towards homelessness dating back to the Poor Laws (Kennett, 2003; Meers, 2012). Thus, UK legal and policy responses to homelessness prioritise 'vulnerability' and unintentional homelessness, including 'natural disasters'. The Act does shape responses to homelessness as a social and civic responsibility. However, it makes no mention of intersecting 'vulnerabilities' or social inequalities.

In Australia, the Australian Bureau of Statistics (ABS) defines homelessness as:

> When a person does not have suitable accommodation alternatives they are considered homeless if their current living arrangement: is in a dwelling that is inadequate; or has no tenure, or if their initial tenure is short and not extendable; or does not allow them to have control of, and access to space for social relations.
>
> (ABS, 2012)

This definition covers adequacy of the dwelling, security of tenure and control of and social access to spaces within a house (ABS, 2012). This aligns with definitions of 'home' in Anglo American and European interpretations that highlight a sense of security, stability, privacy, safety and the ability to control one's living space (Mallett, 2004). However, a person who is experiencing domestic violence and remains in their unsafe home with the perpetrator tends not to be considered homeless because of the difficulties measuring these circumstances (ABS, 2012). This definition also makes no mention of intersecting social inequalities and social processes that contribute to homelessness.

Tiered or pathway definitions of homelessness are influential in Australia, and include Chamberlain's (1999) primary, secondary, tertiary and marginal categories of homelessness. Primary (or literal) homelessness is akin to 'rough sleepers' or rooflessness. Secondary homelessness includes people with no place of usual residence (such as 'couch surfing' or living in temporary shelters). Tertiary homelessness includes people who are inappropriately or insecurely housed, living in culturally defined substandard accommodation. Marginal housing refers to people who are 'at risk' of homelessness, such as those living in boarding houses, being in financial housing crisis or overcrowding. These policy representations of homelessness imply a pathways approach, a linear progression and a continuum of homelessness. The solution to homelessness is represented as 'suitable' housing and homeownership is assumed to be the most desired outcome of housing policies. There is some mention of Aboriginal and Torres Strait Islander experiences of homelessness (ABS, 2012) but nothing about *intersecting* social discriminations.

Similarly, the European Typology of Homelessness and Housing Exclusion (ETHOS) also defines homelessness on a continuum of roofless to inadequate housing (Amore *et al.*, 2011). ETHOS defines homelessness as: roofless, houseless, insecure, inadequate and temporary housing, such as mobile homes. The ETHOS conceptual model was developed by housing scholars Joe Doherty, Bill Edgar and Hank Meert to include social, physical and legal domains of housing and home (Doherty *et al.*, 2004; Amore *et al.*, 2011). This definition has been noted to not always be measurable, and only focusing on places of habitation at one point in time, and not on environmental circum-stances (Amore *et al.*, 2011).

In New Zealand (NZ), housing and health scholars Amore *et al.* (2011, pp. 22–23) argued that homelessness definitions need to consider: cultural, institutionalised and governance contexts, conceptualisations regarding how to measure categories, operational aspects that relate to the 'real world', such as measuring homelessness prevalence, incidence and over the lifetime, as well as whether there is a system that makes measuring homelessness possible, practical, acceptable and affordable. The New Zealand definition of home-lessness refers to 'living in a place of habitation that is below a minimum adequacy standard' and 'lacking access to adequate housing', which are inter-sected with social, physical and legal domains of home (Amore *et al.*, 2011, p. 32). For example, having no accommodation would fulfil the criteria of 'physically inadequate, socially inadequate, and legally insecure living situa-tions'; temporary accommodation would be 'socially inadequate and legally insecure living situations'; sharing accommodation with friends or family would be 'physically inadequate and legally insecure living situations'; and 'uninhabitable housing' would be 'physically and socially inadequate living situations' (Amore *et al.*, 2011, p. 33). Therefore, the NZ definition builds on the ETHOS definition by intersecting social, physical and legal domains with different housing circumstances.

Nonetheless, statutory definitions in the USA, UK, Australia, NZ and the EU all imply that homelessness is the lack of housing, thereby constructing homelessness as a housing problem. These definitions of homelessness do aim to reduce housing inequalities and promote housing justice. However, such definitions measure homelessness according to normative housing catego-ries and assume that 'home' or housing is a safe place (Tomas and Dittmar, 1995, p. 493). Assumptions that housing is the solution and homelessness is the problem do not always acknowledge diverse and contested meanings and experiences of home and homelessness (Somerville, 1992; 2013). Left unex-amined are the broader political debates about the intersecting contributors to homelessness. For example, how do classing, gendering, racialising and heteronormative policy-making processes intersect and shape homelessness? This reflexive attention to power relations in the policy-making process is cen-tral to intersectional policy making and social work.

It has also been noted that the existence of homelessness is a consequence of how housing policies are failing to cope with social and economic changes to the housing and labour markets. What is invisible in these definitions of homelessness is that social housing has been a low priority for many govern-ments, who tend to favour homeownership policies. Yet homeownership is unachievable for many disadvantaged people. Certainly, the housing policies of different countries vary. However, there is insufficient space in this book on homelessness to discuss the housing policies in each country in the EU and each state in the US, particularly as they are aligned to different wel-fare systems (see other books, for example, Balchin, 1996; Schwartz, 2015).

In Australia, homeownership (along with employment) has been the 'corner-stone of the Australian welfare state' but increasing house prices to income ratios has decreased housing affordability (Carson and Kerr, 2014, p. 194). Housing trends influenced by neoliberal market reforms to the welfare state have reduced the availability of public and affordable housing (Carson and Kerr, 2014). Government policies have curtailed the funding of public hous-ing, average house prices have increased relative to income, average monthly repayments on home loans have increased, the proportion of first homebuy-ers has fallen and there is increasing competition for housing in the private rental market, where landlords exercise considerable discretion in choice of tenant (SACOSS, 2007, p. 79). Moreover the Indigenous household rate of homeownership is one-third compared to two-thirds of non-Indigenous households (AIHW, 2011). These housing trends also affect women because of their lower income, inequalities in the labour market and the 'gender pay gap' (ABS, 2014). Home ownership is lower for female *sole* parents (41 per cent) than male *sole* parents (50 per cent) and more men (80 per cent) than women (74 per cent) over the age of 75 years own their home outright (ABS, 2013). These statistics enable social workers to question who benefits and who loses in the implementation of housing, homeownership and homeless-ness policies. My argument is that an intersectional analysis can contribute to understanding how intersecting social and housing disadvantages continue to be maintained, including by favouring homeownership policies.

Typically, social workers are employed within a residual model of welfare involved in providing services to the most disadvantaged and to meeting peo-ple's 'basic needs' (Zufferey, 2008; Carson and Kerr, 2014, p. 11). Within these different welfare state constraints, it remains important for social workers to ask questions about how standardised policies can address the specific conse-quences of oppression for different disadvantaged groups, especially if inter-sections are not specified in social policies (Bishwakarma *et al.*, 2007, p. 34). The next section focuses on Housing First policy formulation and implemen-tation and asks questions about how proposed policy solutions reduce social inequalities and promote social justice.

Policy formulation and implementation of Housing First

As Hankivsky (2012b) and Bishwakarma *et al.* (2007, p. 29) note, the following two questions are fundamental in policy formulation: What kind of programme/policy is envisioned? What are the desired or intended results? After identifying and researching the problem, policy formulation identifies options for intervention that are politically, socially and economically influenced (Carson and Kerr, 2014, p. 87). Currently, the favoured homelessness policy initiatives in Europe, Canada, USA and Australia relate to 'housing the homeless', such as through 'Housing First' approaches.

The formulation and implementation of Housing First initiatives that aim to provide permanent accommodation and support services for the chronically homeless, align with assumptions in statutory definitions of homelessness that represent the problem of homelessness as a lack of housing, caused by chronic disabilities. Social work authors from the USA Deborah Padgett, Benjamin Henwood and Sam Tsemberis have thoroughly examined Housing First (HF) in their new book, which includes a chapter of personal stories of individuals who experienced HF. They trace the 'homeless industry' of shelters, not for profit, religious and philanthropic organisations and advocacy groups, and the story of Housing First that resisted dominant ideas such as treatment first, sobriety and housing readiness (Padgett *et al.*, 2015). The formulation of Housing First included fundamental principles such as: consumer choice, harm reduction, immediate access to permanent independent housing in the community, that housing is a basic human right, client self-determination, respect, a commitment to working with clients for as long as they need, independent apartments, the separation of housing and treatment services, and a recovery orientation (Tsemberis, 2010; Padgett *et al.*, 2015). The policy intentions of Housing First approaches were to permanently house and support an individual according to their individual 'needs and preferences' (Benjaminsen, 2014, p. 12). Housing First principles are also seen to be positive and consistent with social work ethics and values (Benjaminsen, 2014).

Housing First approaches have been implemented and transferred across the Western world. The Housing First pathway models taken up in the UK and Europe were developed by Beyond Shelter Inc. in 1988 in Los Angeles and Pathways to Housing in New York in 1990 (Tsemberis, 2010). The Housing First approach was promoted as an alternative to 'treatment first' (such as for mental illness), the 'housing care continuum' and transitional responses to homelessness, such as commencing from the 'streets' to crisis services and emergency shelters, to transitional housing and then 'independent living'. In Canada, the five year 'At Home/Chez Soi' project was launched in five cities (2009–2013), each with a particular area of focus: Vancouver concentrated on people also experiencing problematic substance use; Winnipeg responded to the urban Aboriginal population; Toronto gave particular attention to ethnoracialised populations, including new immigrants who do not speak English; Montréal included a vocational study; and Moncton provided a smaller city community service. This Canadian response illustrates the flexibility of Housing First.

The Housing First emphasis has also influenced the EU response to homelessness, especially since the European Parliament passed a written declaration on ending homelessness in 2007. Called the 'Housing First Europe' project, the model was trialled in 10 European cities (Amsterdam, Budapest, Copenhagen, Glasgow, Lisbon, Dublin, Ghent, Gothenburg, Helsinki and Vienna) from August 2011 to July 2013 (Benjaminsen and Dyb, 2010; Benjaminsen, 2014). Following the same principles as the Canadian and American projects, in 2010, the French government launched a Housing First programme in Paris, Toulouse, Marseille and Lille called 'Un Chez-Soi d'abord', focusing on people with mental illness or drug and alcohol addictions.

The supportive accommodation model taken up in Australia, called Common Ground, was founded in Time Square, New York City in the 1990s with the aim of ending chronic homelessness (Parsell *et al.*, 2014). This approach has had a massive and rapid uptake across Australia, involving building inner city apartments for people who are homeless and providing intensive support. In the implementation process, 'professional intuition and personal experience were afforded a higher status than formal evaluative evidence' (Parsell *et al.*, 2014, p. 69). Promoted in the national government's homelessness policy *The Road Home* (2008), Housing First aims to increase the supply of affordable housing as central to reducing homelessness (Australian Government, 2008). However, even these Housing First-focused approaches have been criticised for being 'one size fits all' approaches that predominantly address housing and do not address other intersecting, structural oppressions that contribute to poverty and homelessness (Stanhope and Dunn, 2011).

In Australia, alongside Housing First responses (such as Common Ground) 'assertive outreach' initiatives have emerged that reach out to 'rough sleepers' to move them into housing. However, it is important to consider whose voices are missing in policies and responses aimed to move people from 'the streets' to 'house the homeless' (Zufferey and Chung, 2006). For example, Indigenous people are being displaced from their land and inner city meeting places where they have significant spiritual connections. Indeed, the perspectives of Indigenous Australians and land ownership debates are rarely considered in policy-making processes about homelessness (Zufferey and Kerr, 2004). This raises questions about whose perspectives are being heard and privileged, which has implications for how well a particular policy or programme has been implemented and how appropriate the actual policy approach is, and for whom? (Bishwakarma *et al.*, 2007, p. 39; Hankivsky, 2012b).

Evaluations of Housing First

Despite the rapid spread of Housing First and associated services, no single policy initiative will be appropriate for all people who experience homelessness. Policy evaluations can identify which approach is most effective and for whom. What is to be evaluated, by whom, when and how, is ideally decided during the policy formulation stage (Carson and Kerr, 2014, p. 89). However, policy and programme evaluation is often an 'after thought' and rarely includes service user-led evaluations (Coltman *et al.*, 2015).

There have been numerous quantitative and qualitative evaluations of Housing First, including in the field of social work, that intersect predetermined variables, such as substance abuse and mental illness with housing success (Tsemberis and Eisenberg, 2000; Culhane *et al.*, 2002; Padgett *et al.*, 2006; 2011). Over 40 cities across America have now demonstrated cost savings using Housing First (Stanhope and Dunn, 2011). In addition to being the 'most cost-effective', Housing First approaches are promoted as the 'most humane approach of providing housing' (Culhane, 2008; McLaughlin, 2011, p. 410). Social work research has documented the subjective experiences and voices of service users and providers in these homelessness programmes (Padgett, 2007; Padgett *et al.*, 2008; Padgett *et al.*, 2011). However, Stanhope and Dunn (2011) note that Housing First was compelling to conservative governments because of the reductionist, narrow and de-contextualised nature of positivist research evaluations that reflected residual approaches to social welfare in the US and the UK (Esping-Anderson, 1990). The evaluations categorised, identified specific needs, and calculated financial costs of not addressing these needs (Stanhope and Dunn, 2011). However, they did not examine intersecting power relations and social inequalities that contributed to and maintained homelessness. Furthermore, the main implementation challenges for most Housing First projects in Europe continue to involve 'securing rapid access to housing', long waiting lists for social housing and overcoming 'stigmatisation, social isolation, poverty and unemployment' (Busch-Geertsema, 2014, p. 25).

Nonetheless, positive programme and research innovations have emerged from Housing First homelessness policy developments, that include inclusive and participatory approaches, such as service user-led evaluations in Canada (Coltman *et al.*, 2015). The Toronto Housing First site houses people with a mental illness and works collaboratively with 'The People With Lived Experience Caucus', to provide a lived experience perspective and advice to the service, by people who have experienced homelessness and used the mental health system (Coltman *et al.*, 2015). This research is discussed in greater depth in Chapter 6.

Furthermore, Fischer (2003) proposes that policy analysts are potentially facilitators of inclusive policy making, if the production of knowledge becomes accessible to all. Thus, citizen inquiries can provide alternative evaluations of homelessness policy. That is, citizens can identify their 'own interests, reframe arguments, make their own decisions', deconstruct policy arguments and highlight relationships of power (Stanhope and Dunn, 2011, p. 281). This participatory style of policy analysis asks the question: What is good for democratic society? (Mayer *et al.*, 2004). In the field of disability, for example, Meekosha (2006) argued that feminist intersectional activists have failed to examine citizenship and disability. She provided an analysis of race, ethnicity, gender and disability, drawing attention to the power of the social processes of naming and classifying 'who does and who does not constitute a full citizen', in regards to the intersecting social constructions of exclusion based on disability (Meekosha, 2006, p. 172). Alternative policy articulations focusing on an inclusionary citizenship (Lister, 2003) promotes participatory access to all citizens, regardless of ability, race, gender, religious affiliation and socio-economic status. When considering an intersectional social work approach, participatory and service user-led evaluations can enhance social work practice and policy responses to homelessness.

Multi-strand approach

With the intent to institutionalise intersectional policy responses and to address diverse and intersecting discriminations, Hankivsky and Cormier (2011) endorse Parken's (2010) Multi-Strand Method as an example of an innovative intersectional policy-making process, which emphasises multiple inequalities. The Multi-Strand Project (Parken and Young, 2007; 2008; Parken, 2010) was developed in the UK in the context of Article 13 of the EU Treaty of Amsterdam (1999), which necessitates that member states must protect citizens from discrimination on 'a number of grounds including gender, race or ethnic origin, religion or belief, disability, age, and sexual orientation' (Hankivsky and Cormier, 2011, p. 223). In 2006, the United Kingdom passed the Equality Act and in 2007 set up the Equality and Human Rights Commission, to oversee 'a full spectrum of inequalities' (Hankivsky and Cormier, 2011, p. 223).The Multi-Strand Project responds to the 'six-strand' equality legislation, which covers gender, disability, race, sexual orientation, age and religion. Hankivsky and Cormier (2011, p. 220) argued that the UK is 'prompting progressive work to develop policy models that are able to address multiple grounds of inequality'. These policy developments that intersect inequalities can potentially involve social workers and also inform policy responses to homelessness.

Hankivsky and Cormier (2011, p. 224) discuss the following four distinct stages of the Multi-Strand Model in great depth: mapping, visioning, road testing and monitoring, and evaluation. This 'equality mainstreaming' process commences with an Evidence Panel of 'experts' (potentially including service users) from key organisations with human rights, equality and policy knowledge, and a vested interest in one or more strands. First, the mapping process involves scrutinising the policy field (such as social care), and asking questions, such as

> Who is it for? What are the intended outcomes? How is the field structured to perpetuate disadvantage? Does the field promote values of dignity, respect and autonomy? How does the policy operate? What are the human right areas? and Who are the stakeholders?
>
> (Parken and Young, 2007; Hankivsky and Cormier, 2011, p. 224)

Next, the mapping also involves gathering information (such as qualitative and quantitative research data from secondary sources), examining current policies and reviewing previous research findings about each equality strand, within the field of social care. The mapped information is then collated into 'vision' changes for the government/s and service provider implementation, and is 'road tested' in diverse scenarios. For example, will the policy work for a gay disabled man living in a rural area, as well as an Indian single mother on a low income? What services need to be in place to enable access? This mapping involves consultation with a diverse range of stakeholders, including service providers, service users, activist and interested groups, about whether changes will have the 'intended benefits' (Parken and Young, 2007; 2008; Hankivsky and Cormier, 2011, p. 224). The last stage, 'monitoring and evaluation', sets equality and human rights outcomes, provides criteria for 'inspectors' who will monitor the achievement of these targets, develops a strategy for the continuing monitoring of achievements, and reviews and changes policies within ongoing feedback loops (Parken and Young, 2007; 2008; Hankivsky and Cormier, 2011, p. 224).

The multi-strand UK intersectional approach connects social policy to diversity, equality and human rights initiatives, focusing on macro (structural) as well as micro (everyday) social change. Murphy *et al.* (2009, p. 62) also call for the examination of interconnecting and reinforcing power relations at the macro (social structures), mezzo (institutions and organisations) and micro (everyday interaction) levels, at different stages of policy making. Consideration of these multilayered macro-mezzo-micro practices that contribute to enhancing social justice and reducing inequalities, are particularly relevant to social work practice. As May (2015, p. vii) notes, an intersectional approach includes 'unsettling' dominant assumptions, examining gaps and silences and rethinking 'how we approach liberation politics.' This emancipatory way of thinking can also apply to social work responses to homelessness. Future directions in homelessness policy making can include intersectional theorising that incorporates an analysis of power relations, examines social justice ethics and principles, acknowledges changing social contexts, geographical locations and diverse service user perspectives, and promotes inclusive and collaborative policy, research and practice.

Conclusion

Policy makers and researchers (including social workers) are involved in advocating for challenging injustices and negotiating meanings with decision makers and others stakeholders in the policy-making process, such as service providers and service users. This includes collaboratively defining the problem (such as homelessness), setting the policy agenda, adopting, implementing, delivering and evaluating policy (Murphy *et al.*, 2009, pp. 59–60). Social workers play an important role in advocating for policy, system and social change, to prevent and end homelessness, and to intervene to assist people who are at risk of and are experiencing homelessness.

The social work purpose involves advocating for making visible intersecting inequalities, even within conservative political contexts that continue to uphold the status quo. Social workers can be involved in: challenging intersecting and disadvantaging categorisations of people (including making visible the diversity of people labelled as 'the homeless'); naming the disempowering effects of social policies, such as on Indigenous communities that have contributed to experiences of 'spiritual homelessness' (Keys Young, 1998); highlighting intersecting inequalities that act as structural barriers to accessing housing; and making visible diverse definitions of home and homelessness, by noting missing voices in social policy development and analysis.

Housing is a basic human right. Responding to human rights violations, the social inclusion of refugees, asylum seekers and cross country migrants are major global policy issues. Depending on the context of each country, social workers responding to homelessness could be working with Gypsy, Roma and other traveller families and communities, refugees, asylum seekers and forced migrants. Therefore, social work responses to homelessness would incorporate knowledge of civil rights and immigration legislation that focuses on 'guaranteeing the rights' of migrants and refugees (Bezunartea-Barrio, 2014, p. 15). However, one of the limitations to making universal claims about human rights and access to housing in responding to homelessness is that policy approaches differ according to localised contexts. For example, one suggestion we made when researching home and homelessness in two remote Australian towns was supporting and resourcing [Indigenous] 'town camps', to address the diverse needs of all people in these communities (Zufferey and Chung, 2015, p. 21). However, these suggestions about 'town camps' are unlikely to be as relevant in, for example, middle-class urban geographical locations, where there are no 'town camps'. This highlights how classed and racialised differences shape understandings of homelessness and intersect with remote, rural and/or urban localities (Cloke *et al.*, 2007). A challenge for social work policy makers involves acknowledging complexity, diversity and the intersections between social locations that are both globally and locally relevant (Yuval-Davis, 2006, p. 205).

I have previously argued that policy definitions of homelessness have tended to marginalise diverse understandings of home and homelessness by categorising and homogenising population groups according to housing 'need', which can reinforce deep-seated community values that maintain unequal gender, class and racialised power relations (Zufferey, 2015). Social workers, as social actors, are called upon in the social welfare struggle to challenge 'androcentric' and sexist interpretations of women's and men's needs, and to question how these needs get interpreted (Fraser, 1989, p. 157). An intersectional social work approach takes this further, to explore how gender intersects with classed and racialised power inequalities, to name a few. For example, social work and social policy advocates can highlight the persistence of poverty and how neoliberal welfare states have failed to address ageism, sexism and racism (Adams, 2002; Cunningham and Cunningham, 2012). Therefore, intersectionality can create spaces for policy challenges and social change, which are never fixed and always 'becoming' (Bacchi and Eveline, 2010). However, social policies themselves are also gendering, racialising, heteronorming, classing, disabling and third-world-making practices that have constitutive, discursive, subjectification and lived experience effects on people governed by these policies (Bacchi, 1999; 2009).

In this chapter, I have shown how the Intersectionality-Based Policy Analysis framework (IBPA) is useful to explore the 'doing' of intersectionality in policy research, activism and practice (Hankivsky, 2012b, pp. 35–38). This policy analysis framework takes into account social justice and intersecting factors that constitute social inequalities, advocates for self-reflexivity and gives voice to diverse knowledge/s. Intersectional analyses can focus on the policy-making process, outcomes of policies and on the privileges of the policy maker. However, the challenging aspect of an intersectional analysis approach is for social workers to examine policy ideas as problem representations and to reflect on their origins, purposes and effects (Bacchi, 2009). This reflexivity acknowledges that social workers are immersed in constructing as well as resisting dominant policy representations. To subject representations of 'social problems' such as homelessness to critical analyses involves examining deeply ingrained assumptions in Western culture, from which no-one is exempt (Bacchi, 2009, p. xix). As social workers, it is important to interrogate our own assumptions about homelessness and 'homeless people' as well as reflect on our own social locations. In the next chapter I further discuss social work practices in the field of homelessness, from this reflexive intersectional social work approach.

Note

1 Hankivsky (2012b) notes that the IBPA questions have been informed by a diverse range of authors, including Abelson *et al.* (2008), Bacchi (1999), Hancock (2007), Hankivsky and Cormier (2009), Harris *et al.* (2007), Parken (2010), Parken and Young (2007), Signal *et al.* (2008), Urbanek (2009) and Weber and Parra-Medina (2003).

References

Abelson, J., Giacomini, M., Lavis, J., Eyles, J. with Thistlethwaite, J., Grace, D. and Shanmuganathan, S. (2008). *Field of dreams: Strengthening health policy scholarship in Canada*. Centre for Health Economics and Policy Analysis (CHEPA) Working Paper Series. Accessed 3 August 2016. www.chepa.org/docs/working-papers/chepa-wp-08-06.pdf?sfvrsn=2.

Adams, R. (2002). *Social policy for social work*. Houndmills, UK: Palgrave.

Amore, K., Baker, M. and Howden-Chapman, P. (2011). The ETHOS definition and classification of homelessness: An analysis. *European Journal of Homelessness*, 5(2), 19–37.

Australian Bureau of Statistics (ABS). (2012). *A statistical definition of homelessness: Information paper*. Cat. No. 4922.0. Canberra, ACT: ABS.

Australian Bureau of Statistics (ABS). (2013). *Gender indicators: Housing circumstances*. Cat. No. 4125.0. Canberra, ACT: ABS.

Australian Bureau of Statistics (ABS). (2014). *Average weekly earnings, Australia*, May 2014. Cat. No. 6302.0. Canberra, ACT: ABS.

Australian Government. (2008). *The road home: A national approach to reducing homelessness*. Canberra, ACT: Department of Families, Community Services and Indigenous Affairs.

Australian Institute of Health and Welfare (AIHW). (2011). *Housing and homelessness services: Access for Aboriginal and Torres Strait Islander people*. Cat. no. HOU 237. Canberra, ACT: AIHW.

Bacchi, C. (1999). *Women, policy and politics: The construction of policy problems*. Los Angeles, CA: Sage Publications.

Bacchi, C. (2009). *Analysing policy: What's the problem represented to be?* Sydney: Pearson.

Bacchi, C. and Eveline, J. (2010). *Mainstreaming politics: Gendering practices and feminist theory*. Adelaide, SA: The University of Adelaide Press.

Balchin, P. (1996). *Housing policy in Europe* (1st ed.). London: Routledge.

Benjaminsen, L. (2014). 'Mindshift' and social work methods in a large-scale Housing First programme in Denmark. (pp. 12–13). In *FEANTSA Magazine: Social work in services with homeless people in a changing European social and political context*. Brussels: European Federation of National Organisations Working with the Homeless (AISBL).

Benjaminsen, L. and Dyb, E. (2010). Homelessness strategies and innovations. (pp. 123–142). In E. O'Sullivan, V. Busch-Geertsema, D. Quilgars and N. Pleace (Eds). *Homelessness research in Europe*. Brussels: FEANTSA.

Bezunartea-Barrio, P. (2014). Social workers: Challenges and contributions to Housing First support programmes. (pp. 14–15). In *FEANTSA Magazine: Social work in services with homeless people in a changing European social and political context*. Brussels: European Federation of National Organisations Working with the Homeless (AISBL).

Bishwakarma, R., Hunt, V. and Zajicek, A. (2007). Educating Dalit women: Beyond a one-dimensional policy formulation. *Himalaya, the Journal of the Association for Nepal and Himalayan Studies*, 27(1). Accessed 4 May, 2016. http://digitalcommons.macalester.edu/himalaya/vol27/iss1/5.

Bowie, S.L. and Dopwell, D.M. (2013). Metastressors as barriers to self-sufficiency among TANF reliant African American and Latina women. *Affilia: Journal of Women and Social Work*, 28(2), 177–193.

Busch-Geertsema, V. (2014). Housing First Europe: Results of a European social experimentation project. *European Journal of Homelessness*, 8(1), 13–28.

Carbado, A. (2012). *When blood won't tell: An intra-categorical intersectional framework for understanding the construction of race*, MA Thesis. Los Angeles, CA: University of California.

Carson, E. and Kerr, L. (2014). *Australian social policy and the human services*. Melbourne, Vic: Cambridge University Press.

Chamberlain, C. (1999). *Counting the homeless: Implications for policy development*. Canberra, ACT: Australian Bureau of Statistics.

Charter of Fundamental Rights of the European Union (2000). Solemn Proclamation of the European Parliament, the Commission and the Council of 7 December 2000, OJ 2000 C346/1.

Cloke, P., Johnsen, S. and May, J. (2007). The periphery of care: Emergency services for homeless people in rural areas. *Journal of Rural Studies*, 23, 387–401.

Coltman, L., Gapka, S., Harriott, D., Koo, M., Reid, J. and Zsager, A. (2015). Understanding community integration in a Housing First approach: Toronto at Home/Chez Soi community based research. *Intersectionalities: A Global Journal of Social Work Analysis, Research, Polity and Practice*, 4(2). Accessed 14 July 2016. http://journals.library.mun.ca/ojs/index.php/IJ/article/view/862.

Crenshaw, K. (1991). Mapping the margins: Intersectionality, identity politics, and violence against women of color. *Stanford Law Review*, 43,1241–1299.

Crowson, N.J. (2012). Revisiting the 1977 Housing (Homeless Persons) Act: Westminster, Whitehall, and the homelessness lobby. *Twentieth Century British History*, 24(3), 424–447.

Culhane, D.P. (2008). The cost of homelessness: A perspective from the United States. *European Journal of Homelessness*, 2(1), 97–114.

Culhane, D.P., Metraux, S. and Hadley, T. (2002). Public service reductions associated with placement of homeless persons with severe mental illness in supportive housing. *Housing Policy Debate*, 13(1), 107–163.

Cunningham, J. and Cunningham, S. (2012). *Social policy and social work*. London: Sage.

Doherty, J., Edgar, B. and Meert, H. (2004). *Homelessness research in the European Union*. Brussels: European Observatory on Homelessness.

Dunn, W.N. (1994). *Public policy analysis: An introduction*. Englewood Cliffs, NJ: Prentice Hall.

Esping-Andersen, G. (1990). *The three worlds of welfare capitalism*. Princeton, NJ: Princeton University Press.

Ferree, M.M. (2009). Inequality, intersectionality and the politics of discourse: Framing feminist alliances. (pp. 86–104). In E. Lombardo, P. Meier and M. Verloo (Eds). *The discursive politics of gender equality: Stretching, bending and policymaking*. London and New York, NY: Routledge.

Fischer, F. (2003). *Reframing public policy: Discursive politics and deliberative practices*. New York, NY: Oxford University.

Fitzpatrick, S. and Pleace, N. (2012). The statutory homelessness system in England: A fair and effective rights based model? *Housing Studies*, 27(2), 232–251.

Fraser, N. (1989). *Unruly practices: Power, discourse and gender in contemporary social theory*. Cambridge, UK: Polity Press.

Hancock, A.M. (2007). When multiplication doesn't equal quick addition: Examining intersectionality as a research paradigm. *Perspectives on Politics*, 5(1), 63–78.

Hankivsky, O. (Ed.). (2011). *Health inequities in Canada: Intersectional frameworks and practices*. Vancouver, BC: University of British Columbia Press.

Hankivsky, O. (2012a). Women's health, men's health and gender and health: Implications of intersectionality. *Social Science and Medicine*, 74(11), 1712–1720.

Hankivsky, O. (Ed.). (2012b). *An intersectionality-based policy analysis framework*. Vancouver, BC: Institute for Intersectionality Research and Policy, Simon Fraser University.

Hankivsky, O. and Christoffersen, A. (2008). Intersectionality, social determinants and health services. *Critical Public Health*, 18(3), 1–13.

Hankivsky, O. and Cormier, R. (2009). *Intersectionality: Moving women's health forward*. Vancouver, BC: Women's Health Research Network.

Hankivsky, O. and Cormier, R. (2011). Intersectionality and public policy: Some lessons from existing models. *Political Research Quarterly*, 64(1), 217–229.

Hankivsky, O., Grace, D., Hunting, G., Giesbrecht, M., Fridkin, A., Rudrum, S., Ferlatte, O. and Clark, N. (2014). An intersectionality-based policy analysis framework: Critical reflections on a methodology for advancing equity. *International Journal for Equity in Health*, 13, 119. Accessed 4 May 2016. DOI: 10.1186/s12939-014-0119-x.

Harris, P., Harris-Roxas, B., Harris, E. and Kemp, L. (2007). *Health impact assessment: A practical guide*. Sydney: Centre for Health Equity Training, Research and Evaluation [CHETRE], University of New South Wales.

Homeless Emergency Assistance and Rapid Transition to Housing Act (HEARTH). (2009). Accessed 6 July 2015. www.hudexchange.info/homelessness-assistance/ hearth-act/.

Housing (Homeless Persons) Act. (1977). Section 2. Accessed 6 July 2015. www. legislation.gov.uk/ukpga/1977/48/section/2/enacted.

Hulko, W. (2015). Operationalizing intersectionality in feminist social work research: Reflections and techniques from research with equity seeking groups. (pp. 69–90). In S. Wahab, B. Anderson-Nathe and C. Gringeri (Eds). *Feminisms in Social Work Research*. New York, NY: Routledge.

Jewell, S. (2003). *Survival of the African American family: The institutional impact of U.S. social policy*. Westport, CT: Greenwood Publishing Group.

Kantola, J. (2009). Tackling multiple discrimination: Gender and crosscutting inequalities in Europe. (pp. 15–30). In M. Franken, A. Woorward, A. Cabo and B. Bagilhole (Eds). *Teaching intersectionality: Putting gender at the centre*. Utrecht and Stockholm: ATHENA, University of Utrecht and Cente for Gender Studies, Stockholm University.

Kantola, J. and Nousiainen, K. (2009). Institutionalizing intersectionality in Europe. *International Feminist Journal of Politics*, 11(4), 459–477.

Kennelly, J. and Watt, P. (2011). Sanitizing public space in Olympic host cities: The spatial experiences of marginalized youth in 2010 Vancouver and 2012 London. *Sociology*, 45(5), 765–781.

Kennett, P. (2003). The production of homelessness in Britain: Policies and processes. (pp. 173–190). In M. Izuhara (Ed.). *Comparing social policies: Exploring new perspectives in Britain and Japan*. Bristol, UK: Policy Press.

Keys Young. (1998). *Homelessness in the Aboriginal and Torres Strait Islander context and its possible implications for the Supported Accommodation Assistance Program (SAAP)*. Canberra, ACT: Commonwealth Dept. of Health and Aged Care.

Lister, R. (2003). *Citizenship: Feminist perspectives*. Basingstoke, UK: Palgrave Macmillan.

Lombardo, E. and Verloo, M. (2009). Institutionalizing intersectionality in the European Union? *International Feminist Journal of Politics*, 11(4), 478–495.

Ludvig, A. (2006). Differences between women? Intersecting voices in a female narrative. *European Journal of Women's Studies*, 13(3), 245–258.

McCall, L. (2005). The complexity of intersectionality. *Signs: Journal of Women in Culture and Society*, 30(3), 1771–1800.

McLaughlin, T.C. (2011). Using common themes: Cost-effectiveness of permanent supported housing for people with mental illness. *Research on Social Work Practice*, 21(4), 404–411.

Mallett, S. (2004). Understanding home: A critical review of the literature. *The Sociological Review*, 52, 62–89.

Manuel, T. (2006). Envisioning the possibility for a good life: Exploring the public policy implications of intersectionality theory. *Journal of Women, Politics and Policy*, 28(3–4), 173–203.

Masocha, S. (2015). *Asylum seekers, social work and racism*. Houndmills, UK: Palgrave Macmillan.

May, V.M. (2015). *Pursuing intersectionality: Unsettling dominant imaginaries.* New York, NY: Routledge.

Mayer, I., Bots, P. and van Daalen, E. (2004). Perspectives on policy analysis: A framework for understanding and design. *International Journal of Technology, Policy and Management*, 4(1), 169–191.

Meekosha, H. (2006). What the hell are you? An intercategorical analysis of race, ethnicity, gender and disability in the Australian body politic. *Scandinavian Journal of Disability Research*, 8(2–3), 161–176.

Meers, J. (2012). What is meant by the term 'vulnerable' in the Housing Act 1996, s.189? Is the discretion given to local housing authorities in deciding who is vulnerable too wide? *The Student Journal of Law*, 3. Accessed 4 May 2016. https://sites.google.com/site/349924e64e68f035/issue-3/vulnerable-housing.

Murphy, Y., Hunt V., Zajicek, A.M., Norris, A.N. and Hamilton, L. (2009). *Incorporating intersectionality in social work practice, research, policy, and education.* Washington, DC: National Association of Social Workers (NASW) Press.

Nixon, J. and Humphreys, C. (2010). Marshalling the evidence: Using intersectionality in the domestic violence frame. *Social Politics*, 17(2), 137–158.

Norris, A.N., Zajicek, A. and Murphy-Erby, Y. (2010). Intersectional perspective and rural poverty research: Benefits, challenges and policy implications. *Journal of Poverty*, 14(1), 55–75.

Padgett, D. (2007). There's no place like (a) home: Ontological security among persons with serious mental illness in the United States. *Social Science and Medicine*, 64(9), 1925–1936.

Padgett, D., Gulcur, L. and Tsemberis, S. (2006). Housing First services for people who are homeless with co-occurring serious mental illness and substance abuse. *Research on Social Work Practice*, 16(1), 74–83.

Padgett, D., Henwood, B., Abrams, C. and Davis, A. (2008). Engagement and retention in services among formerly homeless adults with co-occurring mental illness and substance abuse: Voices from margins. *Psychiatric Rehabilitation Journal*, 31(3), 226–233.

Padgett, D., Stanhope, V., Henwood, B. and Stefancic, A. (2011). Substance use outcomes among homeless clients with serious mental illness: Comparing housing first with treatment first programs. *Community Mental Health Journal*, 47(2), 227–232.

Padgett, D., Henwood, B. and Tsemberis, S. (2015). *Housing First: Ending homelessness, transforming systems, and changing lives.* Oxford, UK: Oxford University Press.

Parken, A. (2010). A multi-strand approach to promoting equality and human rights in policymaking. *Policy and Politics*, 38(1), 79–99.

Parken, A. and Young, H. (2007). Integrating the promotion of equality and human rights for all. Unpublished report for the Welsh Assembly Government and Equality and Human Rights Commission. Cardiff, Wales: Towards the Commission of Equality and Human Rights.

Parken, A. and Young, H. (2008). Facilitating cross-strand working. Unpublished report for the Welsh Assembly Government.

Parsell C., Fitzpatrick, S. and Busch-Geertsema, V. (2014). Common Ground in Australia: An object lesson in evidence hierarchies and policy transfer. *Housing Studies*, 29(1), 69–87.

Passaro, J. (1996. Reprint 2014). *The unequal homeless men on the streets, women in their place.* London: Routledge.

Robson, P. and Poustie, M. (1996). *Homeless people and the law*. London: Butterworths.

Rönnblom, M. (2008). Policy, power and space: Towards an intersectionality methodology in policy analysis. Paper presented at the POWER Conference. Tampere, Finland.

Schwartz, A. (2015). *Housing policy in the United States* (3rd ed.). New York, NY: Routledge.

Signal, L., Martin, J., Cram, F. and Robson, B. (2008). *Health equity assessment tool: A user's guide*. Wellington, NZ: New Zealand Ministry of Health.

Somerville, P. (1992). Homelessness and the meaning of home: Rooflessness or rootlessness? *International Journal of Urban and Regional Research*, 16(4), 529–539.

Somerville, P. (2013). Understanding homelessness. *Housing, Theory and Society*, 30(4), 384–415.

South Australian Council of Social Services (SACOSS). (2007). *Blueprint for the eradication of poverty in South Australia*. Adelaide, SA: SACOSS.

Stanhope, V. and Dunn, K. (2011). The curious case of Housing First: The limits of evidence based policy. *International Journal of Law and Psychiatry*, 34, 275–282.

Stevenson, D. (2013). *The city*. Cambridge, UK: Polity Press.

Strid, S., Walby, S. and Armstrong, J. (2013). Intersectionality and multiple inequalities: Visibility in British policy on violence against women. *Social Politics*, 20(4), 558–581.

Tomas, A. and Dittmar, H. (1995). The experience of homeless women: An exploration of housing histories and the meaning of home. *Housing Studies*, 10(4), 493–513.

Tonkiss, F. (2013). *Cities by design. The social life of urban form*. Cambridge, UK: Polity Press.

Tsemberis, S. (2010). *Housing First: The pathways model to end homelessness for people with mental illness and addiction*. Center City, MN: Hazelden.

Tsemberis, S. and Eisenberg, R.F. (2000). Pathways to housing: Support housing for street-dwelling homeless with psychiatric disabilities. *Psychiatric Services*, 51, 487–493.

United Nations General Assembly. (2014). *Report of the Special Rapporteur on violence against women, its causes and consequences, Rashida Manjoo* (pp. 1–21). Geneva: UN.

Urbanek, D. (2009). *Towards a processual intersectional analysis*. Vienna: QUING.

Verloo, M. (2006). Multiple inequalities, intersectionality and the European Union. *European Journal of Women's Studies*, 13(3): 211–228.

Verloo, M., Meier, P., Lauwers, S. and Martens, S. (2012). Putting intersectionality into practice in different configurations of equality architecture: Belgium and the Netherlands. *Social Politics*, 19(4), 513–538.

Weber, L. and Parra-Medina, D. (2003). Intersectionality and women's health: Charting a path to eliminating health disparities. *Advances in Gender Research*, 7, 181–230.

Wilkinson, L. (2003). Advancing a perspective on the intersections of diversity: Challenges for research and social policy. *Canadian Ethnic Studies*, 35, 26–38.

Yuval-Davis, N. (2006). Intersectionality and feminist politics. *European Journal of Women's Studies*, 13(3), 193–209.

Zufferey, C. (2008). Responses to homelessness in Australian cities: Social worker perspectives. *Australian Social Work*, 61(4), 357–371.

Zufferey, C. (2011). Homelessness, social policy, and social work: A way forward. *Australian Social Work*, 64(3), 241–244.

Zufferey, C. (2014). Questioning representations of homelessness in the Australian print media. *Australian Social Work*, 67(4), 525–536.

Zufferey, C. (2015). Intersectional feminism and social work responses to homelessness (pp. 90–103). In S. Wahab, B. Anderson-Nathe and C. Gringeri (Eds). *Feminisms in social work research*. New York, NY: Routledge.

Zufferey, C. (2016). Homelessness and gender. In N. Naples, R. Hoogland, M. Wickramasinghe and A. Wong (Eds). *The Wiley-Blackwell encyclopedia of gender and sexuality studies*. DOI: 10.1002/9781118663219.wbegss010.

Zufferey, C. and Chung, D. (2006). Representations of homelessness in the Australian print media: Some implications for social policy. *Just Policy*, 42, 33–38.

Zufferey, C. and Chung, D. (2015). 'Red dust homelessness': Housing, home and homelessness in remote Australia. *Journal of Rural Studies*, 41, 13–22.

Zufferey, C. and Kerr, L. (2004). Identity and everyday experiences of homelessness: Some implications for social work. *Australian Social Work*, 57(4), 343–353.

Zufferey, C., Chung, D., Franzway, S., Wendt, S. and Moulding, N. (2016). Intimate partner violence and housing: Eroding women's citizenship. *Affilia: Journal of Women and Social Work*. DOI: 10.1177/088610991562621.

5 Social work practice and homelessness

This chapter focuses on social work practice responses to homelessness, commencing with a discussion of social work and homelessness literature in the USA, UK and Australia. Drawing on data from interviews with Australian social workers employed as managers, policy makers and 'frontline' workers, I highlight the complexities of social work responses to homelessness, that social work feminist approaches to homelessness can be broadened to incorporate intersectionality, and that social workers embody unequal and intersecting power relations and social locations that constitute their responses to homelessness. To engage with the reflexive aspects of intersectionality and to illustrate personal and professional tensions for two social workers in this field of practice, I provide my own reflexive commentary and a case study analysis by Dr Chris Horsell. In this chapter, I highlight how an intersectional social work approach can subvert dominant practices and expand social work advocacy, by focusing on intersecting power relations.

Background

The central purpose of social work is to influence social change and redress inequalities (Allan *et al.*, 2003), which also resonates with the social justice aims of intersectionality. Social work ethics involve effectively communicating with diverse population groups, showing warmth, empathy, respect, compassion, respecting people's self-determination, being reflexive, non-judgemental and developing trusting relationships (Bezunartea- Barrio, 2014, p. 15). Social workers are involved in social mobilisation and collective action to advocate against breaches of human rights, including how globally, Indigenous peoples, refugees and migrants are affected by homelessness (Bezunartea-Barrio, 2014, p. 15; Mostowska, 2014). However, homelessness is responded to by social workers within historical policy contexts, organisational imperatives and social institutions that are unequal, multilayered and complex, and that can continue to promote disempowering policies and colonising practises.

The social work and intersectionality literature includes: advocating for teaching intersectionality to students of diverse disciplines at undergraduate and postgraduate levels (Carbin and Edenheim, 2013); using it as a human rights policy frame and incorporating it in social work practice, research, policy and education (Murphy *et al.*, 2009); as a tool for critical reflection in social work for analysing a critical incident (Mattsson, 2014); and as an approach when considering creative research methodologies (Bryant, 2016). Social workers have been criticised for neglecting their activist roots and adapting to the contemporary neoliberal context that promotes individual responsibility (Zufferey, 2008; Gordon and Zufferey, 2013). Therefore, embracing intersectionality in social work practice with people who are homeless would involve re-examining the radical social work agenda and how homelessness and social work are constituted through unequal and intersecting power relations.

Historically, social work responses to poverty were dominated by religious, church-based, charity welfare organisations, including the Charity Organisation Societies (COS) that distributed relief to the poor. Direct service workers were often volunteers who were predominantly white, middle-class women with particular values about class, gender, family, work, age and sexuality, which they tried to impose on the working classes (Abrams, 2000; Cree, 2002, p. 280). Men tended to be in paid leadership positions and managers (Camilleri, 1996), which continues in the contemporary social work workforce. The Settlement Houses (or Movements) took a more community-focused approach, in which workers from the 'educated classes' lived in 'working class communities' and became integrated into the neighbourhood and community life (Camilleri, 1996). This movement emphasised community and state responsibility for sanitation, housing, health care, education, social services and employment. These responses to poverty as the practice origins of social work have shaped the individual-structural tensions discussed in the discipline's literature and its responses to homelessness.

Furthermore, in Western countries, the majority of social workers continue to be of Caucasian background. However, the client population include a disproportionate number of women and ethnic minority groups (Whitaker *et al.*, 2006), including people living in unfit dwellings. When examining homelessness and intersectionality in the USA, Lurie *et al.* (2015) note that discrimination results in disproportionate numbers of racial minority groups, women, people who identify as lesbian, gay, bisexual, transgender, intersex and questioning (LGBTIQ), individuals with a mental illness, formerly incarcerated individuals and veterans being evident in homelessness statistics. As well, similar to the unequal power relations between service users and social workers, the social work profession itself is permeated by intersecting and unequal power relations. For example, despite the Equal Pay Act of 1963 being passed, an National Association of Social Workers (NASW) workforce study notes that a significant gender gap in salaries for licensed social workers continues (Whitaker *et al.*, 2006), which reflects the experiences of social workers in other Western countries. Therefore, the social work workforce itself is constituted by intersectional inequalities and social work practice is imbued by gendered, classed and racialised social relations.

As discussed previously, historically 'social work' with 'the homeless', especially in the USA, was practised by voluntary organisations that predominantly focused on older white males with alcohol problems, living in lodging houses, in 'skid row' areas (Johnson and Cnaan, 1995). After the 1930s, when social workers took a more clinical role, 'serving old hobos' was not deemed a priority (Johnson and Cnaan, 1995). A 'new face' of homelessness was noted in the 1980s that focused on families, children and young women, who were deemed more deserving of assistance (Neale, 1997; Rosenthal, 2000), and were often from ethnic minority groups. More recently, Bowpitt *et al.* (2014, p. 1252) examined homelessness day care services in the UK, and found that they function as both places of refuge and places of change, for the 'undeserving homeless' (often men), who are frequently barred from other services. They argued that contemporary individual and social change efforts to end homelessness resonate with historical individual-structural tensions and dilemmas in social work (Bowpitt *et al.*, 2014).

Early feminist and social work scholars who focused on working with homeless women correctly noted that the feminisation of poverty, shortage of affordable housing, abuse and violence 'will not disappear in the 21st century' (Harris, 1991; Russell, 1991; Johnson and Richards, 1995, p. 248). More recently, social science scholars Mayock *et al.* (2015) documented the biographies of 34 women with lengthy homeless histories in Ireland. They found that women who were homeless at an early age 'typically reported family conflict, parental substance use, and/or violence or abuse in the family home' (Mayock *et al.*, 2015, p. 883). For women who became homeless at a later age, the cause was frequently related to intimate partner violence, whilst for those who were bought up in foster care, they always considered themselves 'homeless' (Mayock *et al.*, 2015). They also found that women depicted emergency hostels as 'compromising' their efforts to escape homelessness, through 'an attempt to regain a sense of themselves' (Mayock *et al.*, 2015, p. 895). This resonates with my Australian research in which I found service users resisted being 'told what to do' in accommodation services (Zufferey and Kerr, 2004, p. 350). This research and its findings are discussed further in the next chapter.

It must be noted that social workers have not always been perceived to be the frontline responders to homelessness. Homelessness is often not deemed desirable work or a priority for social workers because engagement is difficult and the work not seen to be 'therapeutic' (Johnson and Cnaan, 1995), when framed within such social work discourses. In listing occupations that care for the homeless, American psychology and health scholars Shinn and Weitzman (1990) did not identify social work, potentially inferring that the profession's expertise was not required. As well, ways of working with the homeless (including case management) is often not taught in social work schools, and field work placements are often not provided in this area. Moreover, in the UK, social workers in local government authorities did not generally work directly with 'homeless people' because of the eligibility criteria for adult social care. Homeless people in the UK tended to be supported through 'housing support workers' who are mostly unqualified workers based in voluntary agencies, rather than by social workers employed in local authorities. However, the recent focus on ending homelessness in policy priorities and legislation means that social workers have increasingly become involved (Benjaminsen, 2014).

In the USA, the NASW policies do focus on homelessness and intersectionality. From 1996 onwards, the NASW Delegate Assembly had approved and revised policy statements on homelessness (NASW, 2005). This comprehensive policy statement categorised homelessness and noted the importance of including the perspectives of people with 'psychiatric disorders', physical disabilities, women and children affected by domestic violence, children living in shelters needing medical treatment, people employed on little income, single mothers unable to work due to lack of child care, 'runaway youth', rural families who have had to abandon their farms, men who are veterans, people with 'chemical dependencies', refugees, asylum seekers and migrants, individuals excluded due to their criminal history, and people affected by disasters (NASW, 2005, pp. 178–179). The NASW (2005) advocate for long-term solutions to homelessness (such as affordable and adequate housing) and for employing social workers to work actively alongside people who are homeless to create advocacy groups, build collaborations between housing, income and support services, support subsidised housing, organise housing assistance programmes for low income families, provide education and supportive job training, end the cycle of homelessness by focusing on children, expand treatment and supportive services and take political action that supports a 'living wage' (NASW, 2005, pp. 182–183). As well, the Council on Social Work Education (CSWE), which is the US' accrediting body for social work schools, departments and programmes, stated:

> The dimensions of diversity are understood as the intersectionality of multiple factors including age, class, color, culture, disability, ethnicity, gender, gender identity and expression, immigration status, political ideology, race, religion, sex, and sexual orientation.
>
> (CSWE, 2008, pp. 4–5)

This focus in homelessness and intersectionality was not evident in British Association of Social Workers (BASW) or Australian Association of Social Workers (AASW) documents. The AASW accreditation standards do focus on foundational curriculum content in social work education, which include values, attitudes, knowledge and skills required for particular specialisations: child wellbeing, mental health, cross-cultural practice and working with Aboriginal and Torres Strait Islander people and communities (AASW, 2012). These policies mention multiple disadvantaging conditions but not intersectionality.

In regards to legislation in the UK, the implementation of the Care Act 2014 for local authorities now requires the development and review of a care and support plan, including collaborating with other services to address housing and accommodation needs. The general responsibilities of the local authorities in the UK, as defined by the Care Act (2014, p. i), include: focusing on individual well-being, preventing the need for care and support, promoting the integration of care with health and other services, providing information and advice, advocating for diversity and quality in the provision of services and co-operating across services in relation to specific cases. Individuals or families who are homeless (or at risk of homelessness) can potentially be encountered by social workers in all services, including these statutory services.

In Australia, Parsell (2011, pp. 330–339) outlines different outreach models for responding to 'rough sleepers'. Traditional models of outreach provide people with blankets, food and so forth (but not housing). Indigenous-focused outreach emphasises 'return to country' strategies to move Aboriginal people back to their remote communities of origin. Assertive outreach responses (such as 'Street to Home') are aligned with Housing First initiatives and aim to end homelessness, by housing people from the 'streets' to a 'home'. Parsell (2011, p. 339) argues that assertive outreach interventions are 'consistent' with the principles of social work because they involve respect for individual self-determination, as well as a commitment to social justice and collective advocacy, such as advocating for access to affordable housing.

In response to Parsell's article in the *Australian Social Work* journal, Coleman (2012, p. 278) calls for a broader social work response to homelessness that extends beyond advocating for rights to housing:

> In a still prosperous, post-industrial Australia, advocating for the right of people sleeping rough to housing will never be enough. Social work needs to actively engage in advocacy for the right of people who sleep rough to education and training; to income security; to freedom from arbitrary 'move-ons' and detention; to basic amenities; and for their right to be recognised as citizens of dignity and worth equal to that of other citizens.

While Parsell (2012) agrees with Coleman's position about social work, he disagrees on another aspect of the debate, which is about whether social workers should advocate for people to have a 'right to be homeless' or 'sleep rough'. According to Parsell (2012, p. 284):

> Accepting rough sleeping as an inevitability and then focusing energy on the rights of people sleeping rough who are left impoverished and marginalised – rather than directing effort toward enabling them to access housing – is, in my view, a misdirected endeavour that is hard to rationalise on the basis of social work principles.

This debate in the *Australian Social Work* journal illustrates some of the dilemmas for social workers in their research and practice with people who experience homelessness and are 'sleeping rough'. In exploring the role of day centres as a 'sanctuary' in the UK, Bowpitt *et al.* (2014, p. 1252), refer to this as the 'oldest dilemmas of social work: how to facilitate change while respecting people's free agency'.

American sociologists Wasserman and Clair (2010, p. 23) have examined how businesses and government work together to legislate and respond against those who are homeless. These strategies involve physically managing city spaces and promoting particular conceptualisations of the public sphere that encourage middle-class pursuits. Inner city legislation and policies across the world have included criminalising homelessness and banning the 'homeless' from public spaces. This trend surely invokes the question of: who counts as a citizen? Wasserman and Clair (2010) argue that the charitable approach of social services that purportedly aims to get people who are homeless 'off the streets' is viewed as a kinder alternative to business and authoritarian government approaches. Yet, social worker and policy maker conceptions of homelessness do not always resonate with the perspectives of people themselves, as discussed in the next chapter.

Whilst universal social work ethics, values and principles are clearly outlined in numerous Codes of Ethics (BASW, 2002; IFSW, 2005; NASW, 2008; AASW, 2010), their implementation is far more complex, and depends on local contexts and individual subjectivities and preferences (Coleman, 2012; Parsell, 2012). Social work responses to homelessness are constituted by economic, social and political aspects of different countries, as well as organisational contexts within which social workers are employed (Zufferey, 2008). This complexity creates tensions for social workers in responding to homelessness. Nonetheless, an intersectional social work approach aligns with the social work mandate for supporting radical social change, and a person's agency within his/her environment (Murphy *et al.*, 2009; May, 2015). Integrating intersectionality in social work responses to homelessness involves: pursuing self-awareness, promoting individual and social change, understanding dynamic and intersecting social contexts, locations and identities, and developing social work knowledge about social diversity – not limited to gender/sex, race, ethnicity, skin colour, migration, national origin, sexual orientation, age, marital status, political belief, religion, mental, intellectual and physical disabilities (Murphy *et al.*, 2009, p. 43).

Intersectional authors have pointed to the importance of researching all members of society, to question the 'imagined normality' of the majority (Christensen and Jensen, 2012, p. 112). This 'majority inclusive' principle points to the value of examining the discourses and lived experiences of privileged populations (such as social workers) and how these privileges shape daily interactions within unequal power relations (Frankenberg, 1993; Christensen and Jensen, 2012, p. 112). This thinking inspired me to conduct research on the experiences of privileged populations, such as social workers employed in the field of homelessness for my PhD, which I discuss next (Zufferey, 2007), after I had completed my MSW research on service user perspectives (Zufferey and Kerr, 2004), which I discuss in the next chapter. In the spirit of self-reflexivity, the lens is turned inwards, onto social workers themselves.

Social work responses to homelessness

What is social work? Who is a social worker? What is the role of social work in the field of homelessness? As published elsewhere (Zufferey, 2007; 2008; 2009; 2012), I interviewed 39 social workers employed in homeless services (during 2003–2004) in South Australia, Victoria and New South Wales. The roles of the participants included policy developers, managers, advocates and frontline service delivery workers (Zufferey, 2007). Professionally trained, they were all eligible to be members of the Australian Association of Social Workers (AASW) and all worked with people who were defined as homeless. The findings of this study have been reported in more depth in *Australian Social Work* (Zufferey, 2008); *Journal of Social Work* (Zufferey, 2012) and *Affilia: Journal of Women and Social Work* (Zufferey, 2009). However, I briefly discuss this research in this chapter to highlight how social workers construct the complexity of homelessness and advocacy, and how social work is an embodied practice constituted by gendered, classed and cultural differences. In the field of homelessness, social work practice is complex, dynamic and diverse, such that it warrants a more complex response, underpinned by intersectional theorising.

The complexity of homelessness and social work practice

The social workers that I interviewed also noted that homelessness is complex and that people who are homeless have complex needs – yet policy and media representations are often framed simplistically. For example, one participant explained: 'I think people want simplistic answers and look at things in a very unilateral, simplistic way and don't want to deal with those sorts of complexities' (female, 41–50, government service manager). Another participant stated:

> I think people that don't work in the area or even bureaucratic … senior people don't understand the complexity … that whole matrix of events that has led that person to being on the street and feeling like they can't get any assistance, or they don't want assistance.
>
> (female, 41–50, government policy manager)

Whilst not mentioning intersectionality, these quotes refer to how media representations and policy responses to homelessness fail to acknowledge complexity and diversity. The quotes also allude to social work dilemmas and debates about individual-structural causes of and solutions to homelessness that have a long history in literature on social work and homelessness.

From its inception, social work was understood as both 'individualist' and 'structural' (or environmental) with the inherent tensions this divide continues to present for contemporary social workers (Lundy, 2004). While the social workers I interviewed did engage in deconstructing the power relations that constitute individual and systemic/structural/social justice dichotomies (Zufferey, 2008; 2012), they noted that their practices were framed around individuals, as evident in the following participant's quote: 'If you want to make a judgement about what are the fundamental causes of homelessness, it's got very little to do with individuals and yet the focus of our work is always around individuals' (male, 41–50, non-government (NGO) worker). However, this same social worker argued that individualised definitions of social problems were a social construction and failed to acknowledge systemic barriers: 'A construction now ... people have "multiple and complex" problems ... individualize ... the problem is the person's ... it fails to acknowledge ... changing social and economic circumstances ... the response of service systems ... are far more complex and difficult to access' (male 41–50, NGO worker).

These quotes highlight that whilst social workers can argue that responses to homelessness are both individual and structural, in practice, social workers respond primarily to individuals. As well, this social worker noted that the construction that homeless people have 'high and complex needs' ignores unequal social and economic structures, and that service systems are increasingly complex and difficult to access. This resonates with the 'new orthodoxy' of homelessness that complicates understandings of individual and structural disadvantages, when discussing explanations for and responses to homelessness (Pleace, 2000). Building on this, an intersectional social work approach would acknowledge *intersecting* individual and structural (or micro, mezzo and macro) inequalities that contribute to shaping homelessness (Winker and Degele, 2011; Murphy *et al.*, 2009). Furthermore, the social locations of social workers and service users contribute to how homelessness is framed as a social problem and responded to by social workers. Therefore, an intersectional social work approach would acknowledge the complexities of social work practice, by intersecting individual and structural tensions, as well as reflecting on the social locations of social workers and service users, thereby contributing to new understandings of homelessness and social work.

Whilst none of my research participants referred specifically to intersectionality, this combining of individual and structural social work approaches does resonate with multilayered analyses of social structures, constructions of identities and symbolic representations of social issues (Winker and Degele, 2011). Social workers also expressed tensions about balancing their organisational responsibilities as 'gatekeepers' of services, a role that involves excluding those who are less 'deserving', with their social work ethics of advocating for the most disadvantaged. As Payne (2014) notes, 'clients', 'social workers' and the process called 'social work' are socially and historically constructed, within organisational contexts and institutional regimes of power. However, social workers do attempt to challenge and resist institutionalised practices that disadvantage their client groups.

Social work advocacy

Social workers' critical thinking and questioning of dominant ideologies is guided by social work values and ethics that focus on social change and social justice (Mostowska, 2014). How social workers frame homelessness has implications for what interventions are promoted and enacted. In Europe, Polish social geographer Magdalena Mostowska (2014) used an interpretive frame analysis to examine social workers' perspectives when working with homeless migrants in European cities. She found that different countries promote different frames, such as the 'migrant worker' overlaid with an 'exceptional humanitarianism' frame in Copenhagen, in contrast to the 'undisciplined deviant' frame in Dublin (Mostowska, 2014, p. 18). In this discourse analysis of social work interventions, Mostowska argued that the humanitarian frame is less focused on economic efficiency and deviancy, allowing service providers to express professional values and ethics more aligned with their profession (Mostowska, 2014, p. 19). This research highlighted that whilst social workers can engage in 'submissive' strategies that are compliant with state regulations (such as excluding persons from a city shelter with no personal documents and number), they can also engage in 'subversive' strategies that undermine state regulations, such as resisting rigid government regulations and informal co-operation between diverse organisations (Mostowska, 2014, p. 24). For example, in Copenhagen, 'subversive' social work strategies included funding migrant-specific programmes with private funds, campaigning, advocacy and change-focused research (Mostowska, 2014, p. 25).

In my Australian research, I also found that social workers resisted and complied with processes that replicate dominant practices and reinforce unequal power relations (Zufferey, 2008; Mostowska, 2014). The positioning of social workers as having greater power over service users was made overt by the following social worker who said: 'There is an increasing subjugation of client's voices and experiences and greater capacity to access power over homeless people's lives' (male, 41–50, NGO worker). This resisting of dominant power relations by listening to client or service user perspectives is an important consideration in social work advocacy when responding to homelessness. This point is also illustrated by the following participant by reflecting on disempowering practices: 'What do our clients understand and how connected do they feel to us, when we use this very alienating, disempowering and disengaged rhetoric?' (female, 21–30, government worker). Thus, the social work profession has a powerful role in publicly questioning and resisting the impact of unequal power relations on people who experience homelessness, advocating *for* and *with* people experiencing (or 'at risk' of) homelessness (Zufferey, 2008, p. 368). In this book I aim to reinforce the advocacy and social change mandate of the social work profession in order to resist and subvert disrespectful responses to homelessness. However, this book also expands on this, to advocate for making visible *intersecting* social inequalities that contribute to shaping social work responses to homelessness.

Expanding advocacy approaches

Social work responses to homelessness are influenced by particular social work theories, such as strengths-based practice (Krabbenborg *et al.*, 2013), empowerment (Lee, 2013), and feminism when working with women who are homeless. This includes intersectional feminism, in social work and the field of family and domestic violence (Laing and Humphreys, 2013). Feminism as an approach has been described as being 'by, about and for women' (Wahab *et al.*, 2012, p. 459), which is valuable in understanding the experiences of women, and giving voice to people who are marginalised and disadvantaged. This beneficial approach can be further expanded using intersectional research, to examine gendered, racialised, classed, heteronormative, ageist and ableist social work practices, and the experiences of service users in multidimensional ways (Connell, 2002; Pease, 2011).

Twelve out of the 39 social workers in my Australian research advocated for a feminist approach to practice (Zufferey, 2008), particularly by those who were female and who were employed to respond to domestic violence in homeless services for women. As one social worker stated, feminism assists social workers working with women to: 'recognise that we are quite different … there is not one kind of women but we do share similar kinds of oppressions' (female, aged 21–30, government social worker). Women (and their children) who are escaping violence experience fear, shame, poverty, lack of respect, recognition and the loss and destruction of their feelings of connection to a 'safe home', often resulting in homelessness (Zufferey *et al.*, 2016). The feminist perspective did enable a critical examination of how gender and homelessness is responded to by social workers. However, at the time of the interviews, none of the social workers articulated an intersectional feminist approach to homelessness, which can expand on and complicate this feminist analysis.

In regards to intimate partner violence (IPV) and homelessness, our recent large Australian study found that IPV erodes women's citizenship, which includes their access to safe and affordable housing, connections to 'home' and participation in community life (Zufferey *et al.*, 2016). When social workers were advocating for people that they worked with, social work advocacy for social justice and social change was occasionally positioned within a discourse of citizenship: 'A homeless person is basically not seen as important or as valued, than a person with a house, who is seen as a "respectable normal citizen"' (female, 31–40, government worker). Social worker participants argued that a 'houseless' person was perceived by society as less worthy or valued, compared to a person who fulfilled normative housing expectations, such as being homeowners. They said that homeless people were perceived as being 'lesser than' citizens but homeless women in particular were deemed more disadvantaged by masculine notions of citizenship: 'Women certainly are ... the second class citizens ... especially women who are at the edges of society ... homeless women are' (female, 51+, NGO worker). Lister's (2003) notion of gendered citizenship is a useful concept to draw on for social workers, to make comment on gendered inequalities and how women who experience homelessness and violence are further disadvantaged and unfairly socially located. However, an intersectional approach would intersect gender with other potentially disadvantaging social locations around experiences of racism, sexism, classism, nationalism and so forth.

There was some acknowledgement by social workers of the institutionalised sexism and racism that affects Aboriginal populations and new arrival communities. This institutionalised discrimination was emphasised particularly in regards to female refugees from African backgrounds whose temporary immigration visas prevented access to social security support, employment and housing. One example was provided by a social worker who worked with migrant and refugee women: 'The situation of domestic violence, where she is not even registered here as a citizen, who is not entitled to any form of assistance, just falls through every single possible gap you can imagine' (female, 31–40, government service). This quote highlights service gaps for new migrants experiencing domestic violence and homelessness. However, the social work profession has been slow in taking up wider concerns of intersectionality. Social work literature argues that the profession itself is ethnocentric because it is a culturally and historically embedded activity that exists within white institutions, unequal social relations and taken-for-granted dimensions of power (Quinn, 2003; Briskman, 2003; Pease, 2010; Walter *et al.*, 2011). The social workers in this study understood this position but without articulating intersectionality. When I asked them about the influence of their gender, age and cultural background, they discussed their experiences of gendered, classed and racialised practices that were privileging and oppressive. As discussed next, class, gender and cultural backgrounds shape social work practice and these social markers are embodied within practice.

Embodied gendered, classed, cultural backgrounds in social work practice

In my analysis of the interviews, I found that social workers' personal and professional subjectivities were embodied, gendered, classed and racialised, and their responses to homelessness contested (see also Zufferey, 2009). For example, an experienced male social worker of working-class background who was employed in a non-government organisation explained how gender and class influenced his perception of social work:

> Work means that you are developing a whole pile of muscle ... sweating ... digging a hole in the ground. I still have to actually say 'this is work',

sitting in a room where someone is bawling [crying] their eyes out ... [It] is still work – different work. I have to keep telling myself that.

(male, 51+, NGO worker)

This quote illustrates gendered and classed constructions of social work, and also highlights its practice as a form of gendered emotional labour, that requires social workers to show genuine but controlled emotion and empathy towards clients or users of services (Barron and West, 2007; Lupton, 1998). This type of emotional labour, such as listening to someone 'bawling', is often considered to be feminised work, not like 'digging a hole in the ground' as masculinised physical work. This dilemma was not experienced by female social workers who tended to describe social work as a 'calling' that they essentialised as their 'nurturing' and 'compassionate' nature. As one female social worker said: 'I have always been a people's person ... I needed to be in this field ... it is kind of ... what I was meant to do' (female, 21–30, NGO worker).

Social workers openly discussed how gender and power inequalities can function as a normative, invisible form of oppression. Confronting his own sense of masculinised privilege, one male social worker who worked for an advocacy body explained: 'I am not the Other. I am man. I am the norm. I don't experience it... . I am not confronted with it' (male, 31–40, advocacy policy worker). This invisible gendered oppression was also noted by one female government social worker who said: 'The subtleties of [gender] oppression ... you internalise that ... subsequently you start to see that you have been oppressed, but you did not know it at the time' (female, 41–50, government manager). These quotes illustrate that social workers in their practice are also affected by intersecting unequal power relations that shape their gendered and classed perceptions and experiences of power within social work practice. These themes are further discussed in my 2009 journal article in *Affilia: Journal of Women and Social Work*, drawing on Connell's (2002) multidimensional gender relations.

As well as gender and class, 12 out of the 39 social workers interviewed identified that their family were refugees, or had migrated to Australia. One non-government female social worker felt that her own experiences of being 'othered' as a migrant (as a child) assisted her to empathise with her client group: 'I was an outsider when I arrived ... I know about outsiders who are homeless people ... I was abused as a child, as "a wog"' (female, 51+, NGO worker; see also Zufferey, 2015, p. 95). In Australia, the term 'wog' is widely used to racially abuse people who migrated from Europe and the Middle East after the Second World War. From the 1980s this term of abuse has been reclaimed in Australian movies such as *Wogs Out of Work* (1987) or *Wog Boys* (2000) written and acted by comedian Nicholas 'Nick' Giannopoulos. The term 'wog' is now often used to assert ethnic identity and 'wog humor' is popular. However, as Mitchell (1992, p. 2) noted, these racial representations also function to caricature and stereotype the physical appearance, culture, customs, habits and language of men and women from culturally and linguistically diverse groups, as a form of 'colonial discourse' and 'apparatus of power'.

Using an intersectional lens, Mehrotra (2010) argued that social workers in a global context must increasingly incorporate discussions on migration, diaspora, nationality, class, age, gender, ethnicity and citizenship status into their analyses. The material realities of homelessness and feeling 'homeless' are embodied experiences marked by limited citizenship rights and economic, political and social power (Arnold, 2004, p. 122). In relation to homeless women, it is well known that the majority were once victims of domestic violence and this gendered experience intersects with classed and racialised experiences of violence. The most severe and lethal domestic violence occurs disproportionately among low-income women of ethnic minority backgrounds, challenging the mainstream feminist contention that domestic violence (and homelessness) affects all women equally (Sokoloff and Dupont, 2005). Moreover, women with disabilities are often in vulnerable situations where abuse can occur, and encounter more frequent domestic abuse and abuse by people in positions of power, such as health care workers (Lockhart and Danis, 2010).

Social work codes of ethics worldwide emphasise that social workers advocate for and address the impact of oppression, social injustice and human rights violations (Murphy *et al.*, 2009). Social workers in my research explained that their personal and professional experiences of racism or sexism have reinforced their commitments to influencing social change. One woman of Chilean background spoke of her family being refugees because they fought for social justice, and this continues in her life today: 'A big part of my life … fighting for social justice and human rights … helping refugees … doing community work without even being paid … that has continued on' [in work with homeless] (female, 31–40, NGO worker). Therefore, in my research I found that professional social workers' commitments to social justice and advocacy for disadvantaged community groups intersect with personal identities and experiences that are embedded within diverse political, social and cultural histories that constitute social work identities and practices (see also Zufferey, 2015). An intersectional social work approach has enabled me to analyse and deconstruct how intersecting unequal power relations constitute social workers' own embodied experiences.

Intersectionality involves reflecting on social workers' own social locations, including for example, highlighting white race privilege, xenoracism, unequal race relations, ethnicity, gender, class, age, sexuality, ability, religion, political orientation and other social markers. These intersecting differences constitute the practice and advocacy efforts of social workers. However, different service users potentially experience the social locations of social workers and their advocacy efforts differently. An intersectional social work approach can emphasise the importance of responding to diverse, embodied and interrelated inequalities, by also giving due accord to the voices and agency of service users, without losing sight of the structural inequalities that impact on their experiences (see Chapter 6).

Intersectionality can assist social workers to reflect on themselves and their practice in the field of homelessness, as constituted within intersecting and institutionalised power inequalities. However, social work has been slow to take up intersectional theorising and to engage with the difficulties involved in incorporating an intersectional analysis into its practice, especially when working with people who experience homelessness. An intersectional social work approach would include examining multifaceted subjectivities and social structures that contribute to maintaining particular social work privileges as they intersect with multiple intersecting oppressions.

Self-reflexivity

As previously discussed in Chapter 2, the notion of *siting* involves the social worker reflecting on his/her situatedness in time, space, history, body, and the intersecting power differentials in his/her own life (Lykke, 2010). In the spirit of reflexive practice, I am interested in focusing on the processes and practices all social workers engage in that continue to reinforce power relations in the field of homelessness, including my own. An analysis of whiteness and white privilege has often been invisible in social work, in the struggle to incorporate notions of power and diversity (Kemp and Brandwein, 2010). This creates tensions for me as a white social work academic, practising in predominantly white and 'racist' ways, in a country where the majority of the population (including social workers) are white, such as Australia. A self-reflexive intersectional approach acknowledges that social work has been criticised for being dominated by white, Western and middle-class discourses (Leonard, 1997; Moreton-Robinson, 2009). Self-reflexivity includes examining my own privilege/s, as well as my own oppression/s. As a social worker who purports to engage in intersectional scholarship, it is important to also locate myself as a subject of privileging/oppressing forces and to attend to the 'oppression *and* privilege' of my own social location, which includes examining the processes involved in maintaining my own privilege (Hulko, 2009, p. 53). Next, I provide a personal account of my professional and personal engagement with intersectionality; my homelessness practice and research in the Australian welfare system, as well as the privileges and oppressions that constitute my own subjectivity.

I have personally and professionally reflected on social work and my white race privilege working as a white social worker in the child protection context in a previous journal article in *International Social Work* (Zufferey, 2013). As a white social worker in Australia I am ascribed an invisible power and privilege as a member of the dominant cultural group (McIntosh, 1992). I am a middle-aged, middle-class, white woman, a first generation Australian of Swiss background. As a white social worker and academic, white race privilege and professional 'expert' power positions me as a 'situated knower' within a racist society (Moreton-Robinson, 2009). As a white person, there is much that I do not know about and will never know or experience of racism in a racist Western society (Tuana, 2006). Although white privilege is a global phenomenon, my experiences of white privilege are geographically and culturally located in the local Australian context.

Although I did not intentionality design the project as intersectional research, I did begin thinking about the notion of intersectionality in 2001, when completing a MSW research thesis on the perspectives and identities of Aboriginal and non-Aboriginal men and women who experience homelessness in Adelaide, South Australia (see also Zufferey and Kerr, 2004). This research was my initial engagement with how experiences and perceptions of home and homelessness were influenced by diverse racialised, classed and gendered social locations, particularly focusing on the perspectives of Aboriginal Australians. At the time of this research, I was a social work practitioner in the field of homelessness in the inner city of Adelaide, South Australia. My role was to collaborate between government and non-government services to improve responses to homelessness, engage in assertive outreach and assist people who were sleeping in the streets and parklands to exit what is commonly understood as 'rough sleeping' or literal 'homelessness'. People I spoke with who were Aboriginal Australians protested about being asked to 'move on' from their traditional meeting places in the inner Adelaide parklands. As one Aboriginal woman in my research explained, the parklands belong to Aboriginal people, stating: 'find out whose land you're really running your cars on. Whose land is this underneath all your little cement?' (Zufferey and Kerr, 2004, p. 348). This raised considerable tensions for homelessness outreach workers who wanted to be culturally responsive but were politically and organisationally constrained, as they were employed within white institutions funded to move people from the 'streets' to a 'home'. This practice tension has remained with me and guided my thinking about the importance of intersectional social work approaches in the area of homelessness.

Whilst considering that the central aim of social work is to be inclusive of diverse client groups, normative social work practices raised dilemmas for me, about being a white, Western and middle-class social worker intervening in other people's lives. I experienced my own social locations in an emotional and embodied way, which was sustained through interactional and relational processes, including my relationships as a social worker with service users. I often felt outraged and frustrated at the social inequalities that were institutionalised within social structures (such as the rich–poor divide) and service systems, including the lack of access to affordable housing. Since completing my PhD research on social work and homelessness in 2007, I have become increasingly conscious of the intersecting influences of class, gender and cultural inequalities in social work responses to homelessness.

More recently, I have been thinking about my own intersecting experiences of both privilege and oppression, as a woman and a single parent. I have been a single mother by choice for the last 22 years. For the first

18 months of being a parent I was entirely dependent on welfare payments, which situated me within a 'welfare dependent' discourse. For example, I recall incidents when my neighbour, who was a truck driver, asked me to clean his house for money and when I declined the job, he was outraged that I was taking money from the government and not wanting to accept his cleaning 'work'. I did (and still do) try hard to ignore and resist the assumptions made about me as a single mother by neighbours, students I teach, colleagues at work and even family and friends. These ideas about single mothers include that I was (or am) sexually promiscuous, that my son who is from a 'broken home' will live in poverty, be a delinquent, not do as well at school, needs a father figure and will consequently, lack self-esteem or self-control. These societal attitudes about single mothers position me as having an 'epistemically disadvantaged identity' reinforced by knowledge practices and prejudices about my character, intellectual capacity, body and nature (Tuana, 2006). As a consequence of experiencing this, I did feel the pressure to return to work earlier than I would have liked. I did not want to be labelled a 'welfare-dependent mother' and to disadvantage my child economically. This shows how I embodied the assumptions of welfare policies and practices that constitute lone mothers' identities as 'worker citizens' that delegitimise 'mothering as both an activity and social identity' (Pulkingham *et al.*, 2010, p. 280). Consequently, my son spent most of his early life in child care, whilst I built my professional and then, academic career. I dedicate this book to him and the parent I might have been, had I not internalised assumptions that as a single parent I was an invisible mother and immoral citizen (Pulkingham *et al.*, 2010). Therefore, when reflecting on my background as a mother, social work researcher, practitioner and now educator, and drawing on intersectional feminism as a theoretical approach, I conclude that it is important to acknowledge our own intersecting experiences of both privilege and oppression. In recognising our own social positions, we are more able to deconstruct the power relations that constitute diverse social worker–service user relationships, when working with people who experience homelessness.

This reflection on my own narrative is aligned with the constructionist approach to intersectionality that views identity as a (subjective) 'narrative construction' (Prins, 2006, p. 277). I do not intend to 'name' my own privileges and oppression as binaries (Prins, 2006, p. 277), as they change over time and in different contexts. This type of self-reflection would be different for each person who reads this book.

The next case study and reflection was provided my colleague and partner Dr Chris Horsell, pertaining to his professional practice as a white, male social worker, when employed in a homeless men's night shelter. The case study below highlights responses of service users that reflect dominant heteronormative assumptions and homophobic responses towards people who identify as LGBTIQ (including 'youth of color'), as identified in literature (Quintana *et al.*, 2010, p. 27).

Case study: Ian

This case study of Ian provides an illustration of how gender binaries and homophobia are institutionalised in the homelessness service provision system that provides for women or men's only services. This case study offers some insights and reflections on the barriers to human rights and social justice for one transgender person experiencing homelessness in Australia.

Ian is a transgender person from a multiracial background, in his mid-thirties, who identifies as a woman. As will be evident from this case study, there were significant challenges in providing a safe and secure environment for Ian within the current homeless services sector. Officially, he could not be accommodated within services for women but within the men's shelter system, he was particularly vulnerable to abuse.

Ian has been homeless for several years and accesses an inner city homeless men's shelter every eight or nine months for emergency accommodation. The accommodation service was renovated in the early 2000s to provide single rooms for some residents, after many years of dormitory style accommodation. However, shared rooms continue to be the case for approximately half of those adult men who present to the shelter.

Ian usually presented wearing a pink jumpsuit (referred to as 'onesies' in the UK) or floral dress. He wore some makeup – usually eyeliner, and on occasions lipstick. He had platinum blonde hair and more often than not wore a tiara. Ian said he suffered from bouts of depression and attempted suicide several times in his life – but did not seek assistance from mental health services, stating he felt they did not understand him.

Staff at the accommodation service noted that on a number of occasions other residents would taunt Ian about his appearance and sexuality, often to the point of provocation. For the most part Ian was relatively calm but if provoked he would invariably respond with a verbal riposte to provocateurs. This occasionally led to other service users attempting to assault him physically. While every effort was made to seek longer-term accommodation for Ian, staff would often experience systemic barriers founded on rigid gender classification.

While one cannot overly generalise, as a social worker in the homeless sector over a number of years I noticed that many male homeless clients performed a dominant heterosexual masculinity that was proscribed by rigid gender classifications which allowed for minimal, if any, crossing of gender boundaries. Additionally, while workers in the field did not necessarily hold similar views, systemic barriers that reflected heterosexual norms made it difficult to provide an appropriate and safe service response for people such as Ian. For example, there were no homeless services available for transgender people and therefore, no service support referral could be made.

Ian's situation challenged me as a social worker at a number of levels. I found myself at times totalising his 'vulnerable' identity as a transgender person and frequently became over protective in the face of the attitudes of other clients who frequently said that he shouldn't be in the service. His situation led me to think more expansively about structural and systemic causes of homelessness. A structural framework in its most orthodox forms takes on board binary gendered responses to men and women and is thoroughly imbued with masculinist assumptions about home and public space, including in a homeless men's shelter. In my own work with Ian at the men's shelter, I had to reflect carefully on my own assumptions and feelings towards other clients, who in many ways were disenfranchised but with regard to Ian, were blatantly abusive and at times violent.

Ian's situation brought into sharp profile for me long-held views about the limitations of normative masculinist assumptions regarding both the social work client base I worked with and the broader homelessness sector that also constructs rigid gender-oriented services. I often felt angry and at a loss as to what would be best to do, not least because of a lack of service options. I learned to deal with gender ambiguity and relearned some basic social work skills about deep listening and affirmation. Whilst I did aim to challenge normative gender constructions in conversations with workers and clients of the service, and advocate for system change and services that could respond to Ian, this was mostly unsuccessful.

Reflection

This case study points to the problem of integrating and operationalising intersectionality in social work responses to homelessness within service systems that are structurally constructed along rigid gender lines. The challenge for social work practitioners is how to collectively respond to the intersecting inequalities experienced by male, female and transgender clients, within normative socio-political and organisational contexts that construct gender/sex binaries and homogenise social issues. An intersectional approach invites social workers to take into account socially constructed aspects of gender performativity (Butler, 1999), and to consider heteronormative assumptions that disadvantage transgender people such as Ian, within multiple and intersecting power inequalities. The complexity of Ian's homeless experience led Chris, the male social worker working in the men's night shelter, to reconsider traditional masculine assumptions in services and by service providers and service users when responding to homelessness. As stated previously, as Murphy and colleagues (2009) noted, intersectionality provides a systems-focused perspective, consistent with social work's commitment to social justice. To dismantle intersecting social inequalities and to move beyond simply focusing on complexity and diversity (May, 2015), social workers also need to challenge normative sex/gender constructions (Lykke, 2010), and advocate for changes to service systems that can respond more inclusively to Ian's experience. However, as Rowntree (2014) has noted, sexuality and gender constructions are neglected areas of analysis in the field of social work education.

In addition to the lack of social services for transgender people and the invisibility of sexuality in social work education, literature indicates that the 'failure' of 'family and social safety nets' to support LGBTIQ people has 'catastrophic consequences on their economic stability, educational attainment, physical and mental health, economic future, and life expectancy' (Quintana *et al.*, 2010, p. 1). A disproportionate number of young people who experience homelessness are gay, lesbian, bisexual or transgender, have higher rates of victimisation and abuse, and are more likely to be discriminated against, attempt suicide and experience mental health, and drug and alcohol problems – but they are overlooked by the welfare system and systemic responses to homelessness (Quintana *et al.*, 2010). The literature on social work and LGBTIQ people does, however, take an intersectional approach, such as Neill *et al.*'s (2015) edited Canadian book that provides insights into multiple and intersecting identities of LGBTQ people and communities, to inform social work practice in the pursuit of social justice.

Conclusion

An intersectional social work approach is reflexive, holistic, empowering, systems-focused and socially just (Murphy *et al.*, 2009). Intersectionality highlights 'that people belong to more than one social category at the same time' by focusing on 'interactions of different social locations, systems and processes' and investigating 'the significance of any specific combination of factors' (Hankivsky *et al.*, 2014, p. 13). This approach can expand advocacy in social work and homelessness, to include diverse and previously invisible intersecting inequalities. For example, it can broaden anti-homophobic, anti-racist and feminist activism in the area of homelessness, to be inclusive of other categories of disadvantage such as disability, whilst also acknowledging social workers' positions of power and advantage (Nixon and Humphreys, 2010; Shaikh, 2012).

An intersectional approach can extend social work understandings about social constructions that intersect to constitute social workers' own professional and personal subjectivities. It invites social workers (and other professions) to reflect on their own social locations and to challenge intersecting social inequalities and contribute to social change. Thus, in the context of social work practice responses to homelessness, an intersectional social work approach allows for a more complex, flexible, multilayered analysis of power locations.

Whilst this chapter is related to social work practice specifically, the range of issues that are constructed as underpinning experiences of homelessness, including domestic and family violence, mental health, complex trauma, physical ill health and drug and alcohol issues, are also domains of other professions. Intersectional analysis is not the exclusive domain of one profession, and is equally relevant in the responses of other disciplines involved in the field of homelessness. Therefore, an intersectional social work approach can be multidisciplinary, assisting different professions to work together, for the benefit of people who experience homelessness, and to contribute to the potential of inter-professional practice. This book focuses on social work because this is my profession and expertise, and because intersectionality is neglected in the field of social work and homelessness. The next chapter examines the perspectives of service users and people who have experienced homelessness.

References

Abrams, L.S. (2000). Guardians of virtue: The social reformers and the 'girl problem', 1890–1920. *Social Services Review*, 74(3), 436–452.

Allan, B., Pease, B. and Briskman, L. (Eds). (2003). *Critical social work*. Crows Nest, NSW: Allen and Unwin.

Arnold, K.R. (2004). *Homelessness, citizenship and identity: The uncanniness of late modernity*. Albany, NY: State University Press of New York.

Australian Association of Social Workers (AASW). (2010). *Code of Ethics*. Accessed 10 March 2012. www.aasw.asn.au/document/item/740.

Australian Association of Social Workers (AASW). (2012). *Australian Social Work Education and Accreditation Standards (ASWEAS) (2012), Guideline 1.1: Guidance on essential core curriculum content*. Accessed 4 September 2013. www.aasw.asn.au/whatwedo/social-work-education.

Barron, D. and West, E. (2007). The emotional costs of caring incurred by men and women in the British labour market. *Social Science and Medicine*, 65, 2160–2171.

Benjaminsen, L. (2014). 'Mindshift' and social work methods in a large-scale Housing First programme in Denmark. (pp. 12–13). In *FEANTSA Magazine: Social work in services with homeless people in a changing European social and political context*. Brussels: European Federation of National Organisations working with the Homeless (AISBL).

Bezunartea-Barrio, P. (2014). Social workers: Challenges and contributions to Housing First support programmes. (pp. 14–15). In *FEANTSA Magazine: Social work in services with homeless people in a changing European social and political context*. Brussels: European Federation of National Organisations working with the Homeless (AISBL).

Bowpitt, G., Dwyer, P., Sundin, E. and Weinstein, M. (2014). Places of sanctuary for 'the undeserving'? Homeless people's day centres and the problem of conditionality. *British Journal of Social Work*, 44, 1251–1267.

Briskman, L. (2003). Indigenous Australians: Towards postcolonial social work. (pp. 92–106). In J. Allan, B. Pease and L. Briskman (Eds). *Critical social work*. Crows Nest, NSW: Allen and Unwin.

British Association of Social Workers (BASW). (2002). *The Code of Ethics for Social Work*. Accessed 12 March 2012. http://cdn.basw.co.uk/membership/coe.pdf.

Bryant, L. (2016). Repositioning social work in feminist epistemology, research and praxis. (pp. 82–98). In S. Wendt and N. Moulding (Eds). *Contemporary feminisms in social work practice*. Abingdon, UK: Routledge.

Butler, J. (1999) [1990]. *Gender trouble: Feminism and the subversion of identity*. New York, NY: Routledge.

Camilleri, P.J. (1996). *Re-constructing social work: Exploring social work through talk and text.* Avebury, UK: Ashgate.

Carbin, M. and Edenheim, S. (2013). The intersectional turn in feminist theory: A dream of a common language? *European Journal of Women's Studies*, 20, 233–248.

Care Act. (2014). Chapter 23. Accessed 6 July 2015. www.legislation.gov.uk/ukpga/2014/23/contents/enacted.

Christensen, A. and Jensen, S. (2012). Doing intersectional analysis: Methodological implications for qualitative research. *Nordic Journal of Feminist and Gender Research*, 20(2), 109–125.

Coleman, A. (2012). Context, context, context: A commentary on responding to people sleeping rough: Dilemmas and opportunities for social work (Parsell, 2011). *Australian Social Work*, 65(2), 274–279.

Connell, R.W. (2002). *Gender.* London: Polity Press.

Council on Social Work Education (CSWE). (2008). *Educational policy and accreditation standards.* Alexandria, VA: CSWE.

Cree, V.E. (2002). Social work and society. (pp. 275–287). In M. Davies (Ed.). *Blackwell companion to social work* (2nd ed.). Oxford, UK: Blackwell.

Frankenberg, R. (1993). *White women, race matters: The social construction of whiteness.* Minneapolis, MN: University of Minnesota Press.

Gordon, L. and Zufferey, C. (2013). Working with diversity in a neoliberal environment. *Advances in Social Work and Welfare Education*, 15(1), 20–30.

Hankivsky, O., Grace, D., Hunting, G., Giesbrecht, M., Fridkin, A., Rudrum, S., Ferlatte, O. and Clark, N. (2014). An intersectionality-based policy analysis framework: Critical reflections on a methodology for advancing equity. *International Journal for Equity in Health*, 13, 119. Accessed 4 May 2016. DOI: 10.1186/s12939-014-0119-x.

Harris, M. (1991). *Sisters of the shadow.* Norman, OK: University of Oklahoma.

Hulko, W. (2009). The time- and context-contingent nature of intersectionality and interlocking oppressions. *Affilia: Journal of Women and Social Work*, 24(1), 44–55.

International Federation of Social Workers. (2005). *Ethics in Social Work: Statement of Principles.* Accessed 12 March 2012. http://ifsw.org/policies/code-of-ethics/.

Johnson, A.K. and Cnaan, R.A. (1995). Social work practice with homeless persons: State of the art. *Research on Social Work Practice*, 5(3), 340–382.

Johnson, A. and Richards, R. (1995). *Homeless women and feminist social work practice.* (pp. 232–257). In N. Van Den Bergh (Ed.). Feminist practice in the 21st century. Washington, DC: NASW Press.

Kemp, S. and Brandwein, R. (2010). Feminisms and social work in the United States: An intertwined history. *Affilia: Journal of Women and Social Work*, 25(4), 341–364.

Krabbenborg, M.A., Boersma, S. and Wolf, J.R. (2013). A strengths based method for homeless youth: Effectiveness and fidelity of Houvast. *BMC Public Health*, 13, 359–369.

Laing, L. and Humphreys, C. (2013). *Social work and domestic violence.* London: Sage.

Lee, J. (2013). *The empowerment approach to social work.* New York, NY: Columbia University Press.

Leonard, P. (1997). *Postmodern welfare: Reconstructing an emancipatory project.* London: Sage.

Lister, R. (2003). *Citizenship: Feminist perspectives.* Basingstoke, UK: Palgrave Macmillan.

Lockhart, L. and Danis, F. (Eds). (2010). *Domestic violence: Intersectionality and culturally competent practice*. New York, NY: Columbia University Press.

Lundy, C. (2004). *Social work and social justice: A structural approach to practice*. Toronto, ON: Broadview Press.

Lupton, D. (1998). *The emotional self*. London: Sage.

Lurie, K., Schuster, B. and Rankin, S. (2015). *Discrimination at the margins: The intersectionality of homelessness and other marginalized groups*. Seattle, WA: Seattle University School of Law and Homeless Rights Advocacy Project.

Lykke, N. (2010). *Feminist studies: A guide to intersectional theory, methodology, and writing*. New York, NY: Routledge.

McIntosh, P. (1992). White privilege and male privilege: A personal account of coming to see correspondences through work in women's studies. (pp. 70–81). In M. Anderson and P. Collins (Eds). *Race, class and gender: An anthology*. Belmont, CA: Wadsworth Publishing Company.

Mattsson, T. (2014). Intersectionality as a useful tool: Anti-oppressive social work and critical reflection. *Affilia: Journal of Women and Social Work*, 29(1), 8–17.

May, V.M. (2015). *Pursuing intersectionality: Unsettling dominant imaginaries*. New York, NY: Routledge.

Mayock, P., Sheridan, S. and Parker, S. (2015). 'It's just like we're going around in circles and going back to the same thing …': The dynamics of women's unresolved homelessness. *Housing Studies*, 30(6), 877–900.

Mehrotra, G. (2010). Toward a continuum of intersectionality theorizing for feminist social work scholarship. *Affilia: Journal of Women and Social Work*, 25(4), 417–430.

Mitchell, T. (1992). Wogs still out of work: Australian television comedy as colonial discourse. *Australasian Drama Studies*, 20, 119–133.

Moreton-Robinson, A. (2009). *Talkin' up to the white woman*. St Lucia, QLD: University of Queensland Press.

Mostowska, M. (2014). 'We shouldn't but we do…': Framing the strategies for helping homeless EU migrants in Copenhagen and Dublin. *British Journal of Social Work*, 44(1), 18–34.

Murphy, Y., Hunt, V., Zajicek, A.M., Norris, A.N. and Hamilton, L. (2009). *Incorporating intersectionality in social work practice, research, policy, and education*. Washington, DC: NASW Press.

National Association of Social Workers (NASW). (2005). *Homelessness. Social Work Speaks*. Policy statement approved by the NASW Delegate Authority, August 2005, 178–186.

National Association of Social Workers (NASW). (2008). *Code of Ethics*. Accessed 12 March 2012. www.socialworkers.org/pubs/code/code.asp.

Neale, J. (1997). Homelessness and theory reconsidered. *Housing Studies*, 12(1), 47–61.

Neill, B., Swan, T. and Mule, N. (Eds). (2015). *LGBTQ people and social work: Intersectional perspectives*. Toronto, ON: Canadian Scholars Press.

Nixon, J. and Humphreys, C. (2010). Marshalling the evidence: Using intersectionality in the domestic violence frame. *Social Politics*, 17(2), 137–158.

Parsell, C. (2011). Responding to people sleeping rough: Dilemmas and opportunities for social work. *Australian Social Work*, 64, 330–345.

Parsell, C. (2012). Response to Ann Coleman: Context, context, context: A commentary on responding to people sleeping rough: Dilemmas and opportunities for social work. *Australian Social Work*, 65(2), 280–285.

Payne, M. (2014). *Modern social work theory* (4th ed.). Houndmills, UK: Palgrave Macmillan.

Pease, B. (2010). *Undoing privilege: Unearned advantage in a divided world*. London: Zed Books.

Pease, B. (2011). Men in social work: Challenging or reproducing an unequal gender regime? *Affilia: Journal of Women and Social Work*, 26(4), 406–418.

Pleace, N. (2000). The new consensus, the old consensus and the provision of services for people sleeping rough. *Housing Studies*, 15(4), 581–594.

Prins, B. (2006). Narrative accounts of origins: A blind spot in the intersectional approach? *European Journal of Women's Studies*, 13(3), 277–290.

Pulkingham, J., Fuller, S. and Kershaw, P. (2010). Lone motherhood, welfare reform and active citizen subjectivity. *Critical Social Policy*, 30(2), 267–291.

Quinn, M. (2003). *Immigrants and refugees: Towards anti racist and culturally affirming practices*. (pp. 75–91). In J. Allan, B. Pease and L. Briskman (Eds). Critical social work. Crows Nest, NSW: Allen and Unwin.

Quintana, N.S., Rosenthal, J. and Krehely, J. (2010). *On the streets: The Federal response to gay and transgender homeless youth*. Washington, DC: Centre for American Progress.

Rosenthal, R. (2000). Imaging homelessness and homeless people: Visions and strategies within the movement. *Journal of Social Distress and the Homeless*, 9(2), 111–126.

Rowntree, M. (2014). Making sexuality visible in Australian social work education. *Social Work Education*, 33(3), 353–364.

Russell, B.G. (1991). *Silent sisters: A study of homeless women*. New York, NY: Hemisphere Publishing.

Shaikh, S.S. (2012). Antiracist feminist activism in women's social service organizations: A review of the literature. *Intersectionalities: A Global Journal of Social Work Analysis, Research, Polity, and Practice*, 1, 70–92.

Shinn, M. and Weitzmann, B.C. (1990). Research on homelessness: An introduction. *Journal of Social Issues*, 46, 1–11.

Sokoloff, N. and Dupont, I. (2005). Domestic violence at the intersections of race, class and gender: Challenges and contributions to understanding violence against marginalized women in diverse communities. *Violence Against Women*, 11(1), 38–64.

Tuana, N. (2006). The speculum of ignorance: The women's health movement and epistemologies of ignorance. *Hypatia*, 21(3), 1–19.

Wahab, S., Anderson-Nathe, B. and Gringeri, C. (Eds). (2012). Joining the conversation: Social work contributions to feminist research. (pp. 455–474). In S. Hesse-Biber (Ed.). *Handbook of feminist research: Theory and praxis* (2nd ed.). Thousand Oaks, CA: Sage.

Walter, M., Taylor, S. and Habibis, D. (2011). How white is social work in Australia? *Australian Social Work*, 64(1), 6–19.

Wasserman, J. and Clair, J. (2010). *At home on the street: People, poverty, and a hidden culture of homelessness*. Boulder, CO: Lynne Rienner.

Whitaker, T., Weismiller, T. and Clark, E. (2006). *Assuring the sufficiency of a frontline workforce: A national study of licensed social workers. Executive summary*. Washington, DC: National Association of Social Workers.

Winker, G. and Degele, N. (2011). Intersectionality as multi-level analysis: Dealing with social inequality. *European Journal of Women's Studies*, 18(1), 51–66.

Zufferey, C. (2007). *Homelessness, social work, social policy and the print media in Australian Cities*, Phd Thesis. School of Social Work and Social Policy: University of South Australia.

Zufferey, C. (2008). Responses to homelessness in Australian cities: Social worker perspectives. *Australian Social Work*, 61(4), 357–371.

Zufferey, C. (2009). Making gender visible: Social work responses to homelessness. *Affilia: Journal of Women and Social Work*, 24(4), 382–393.

Zufferey, C. (2012). Jack of all trades, master of none? Social work identity and homelessness in Australian cities. *Journal of Social Work*, 12(5), 510–527.

Zufferey, C. (2013). 'Not knowing that I do not know and not wanting to know': Reflections of a white Australian social worker. *International Social Work*, 56(5), 659–673.

Zufferey, C. (2015). Intersectional feminism and social work responses to homelessness. (pp. 90–103). In S. Wahab, B. Anderson-Nathe and C. Gringeri (Eds). *Feminisms in social work research*. New York, NY: Routledge.

Zufferey, C. and Kerr, L. (2004). Identity and everyday experiences of homelessness: Some implications for social work. *Australian Social Work*, 57(4), 343–353.

Zufferey, C., Chung, D., Franzway, S., Wendt, S. and Moulding, N. (2016). Intimate partner violence and housing: Eroding women's citizenship. *Affilia: Journal of Women and Social Work*. DOI: 10.1177/088610991562621.

6 Lived experiences of homelessness

Introduction

This chapter highlights the diverse 'voices' of service users and people affected by homelessness, including their perceptions of the effectiveness of social work policies and services. I commence this chapter by presenting my original research on the everyday lived experiences of homelessness, from the perspectives of Aboriginal and non-Aboriginal male and female service users in Adelaide, South Australia (Zufferey and Kerr, 2004). Although this research was not initially designed and analysed from an intersectional approach, I centred the voices of people who experienced homelessness, intersected two categories of difference and analysed gendered and race relations. In this chapter I also discuss my research projects on home and homelessness focusing on sexuality, migration, different ethnicities, classes, genders and ages. I draw on insights from research literature about gendered violence and women's homelessness, as well as children's and young people's perspectives of homelessness, as they intersect with gender, race and ethnicity. I argue that the voices of the least powerful are often ignored or re-constructed for particular political purposes. Finally, I highlight service user-led evaluation research (Coltman *et al.*, 2015) as the way forward, to further promote reflexive approaches to social work practice.

Background

Homelessness is a significant and complicated social issue. Homelessness 'stands as a challenge to widely held beliefs about opportunity and success' and it highlights the importance of 'structural obstacles and inequality' in Western societies (Wasserman and Clair, 2010, p. 8). However, 'homelessness is not a characteristic of people but rather a condition in which some people find themselves at some point in time' (Blasi, 1990, p. 209). The perspectives of people who experience homelessness can offer insights into how to begin to think about homelessness in new ways, beyond simply providing solutions on how to end homelessness. They can offer alternative perspectives on policy and service responses to homelessness that acknowledge intersecting complexities and diversity. Wasserman and Clair (2010, p. 2) note that one of the most difficult social problems of our time is the 'us–them dichotomy' view of the world. For example, homelessness is a stigmatised social identity that is given meaning according to its conceptual distance from 'the housing norm' (Wasserman and Clair, 2010). Homogenous representations of and responses to homelessness can limit what can be thought and said about the issue, and dichotomous ways of seeing the world underlie social work practices that continue to maintain unequal power relations. These discourses and practices contribute to shaping the experiences and subjectivities of people experiencing homelessness (Bacchi, 2009; Zufferey, 2014, p. 8). Negative discourses and constructions of homelessness can have pathologising effects on the identities of service users. However, service users can also resist deleterious explanations about homelessness (Zufferey and Kerr, 2004).

In making visible diverse perspectives on homelessness, the concept is shown to be a 'politically contested' rather than objective reality (Fitzpatrick and Christian, 2006, p. 315; Jacobs *et al.*, 1999; Zufferey and Chung, 2015). Whilst there is a widening policy and research understanding of homelessness as outlined in Chapters 3 and 4, few studies focus on intersections in subjective perspectives and embodied lived experiences. Intersectional approaches to homelessness can enable the deconstruction of how unequal social relations intersect and shape the subjectivities of men and women who are defined as homeless. However, I acknowledge that not all social relations that shape the lived experiences of homelessness can be addressed in the chapter. This chapter covers the perspectives of Aboriginal and non-Aboriginal men and women in the Australian context, discusses service user resistances and identifications with negative discourses of homelessness, highlights diverse perspectives on race relations, explores gendered violence and women's homelessness as it intersects with race and ethnic differences, mentions gender and sexuality, covers gender, ethnicity and age differences ranging from children in homeless shelters in the UK to older people in aged care facilities in Australia, and diverse experiences of home and homelessness, including refugees and migrant perspectives. When I reflected on what was missing in this chapter, I noticed that able-bodiedness or disability, nationalism and global-local geographical locations were not explored, which are among numerous other intersecting social locations that contribute to homelessness, and could have been included but were not. As Wasserman and Clair (2010, p. 4) learnt, there is a 'wealth of knowledge on the street that had escaped most of society', even social workers and social services.

The social dynamics of oppression and privilege incorporate a number of dimensions and present individuals (such as social workers) with access to resources and institutional power beyond the advantages of people who do not belong to these groups (Pease, 2010). My dilemmas in this chapter related to the questions: What identity categorisations do I privilege and what do I make invisible? How do I continue to construct and essentialise what inequalities do or do not matter? Who and what contributes to constituting who remains 'at the margins', such as homeless? Who decides who is privileged and who is oppressed? Who benefits from these constructions and decisions? These are difficult questions to answer, but obtaining the diverse perspectives of people being subjected to the identity category of 'homeless' goes some way to making visible the intersecting complexities and diversities of homelessness. As well, social work, with its commitment to social justice and human rights, is an ideal profession for responding to homelessness, in all its iterations. Such social work practice would involve 'activism' that occurs in dialogue with people who have lived experiences of the topics being studied, including service users (Yeatman, 1998).

When analysing a narrative life-interview of one female Bulgarian migrant in Vienna, political scientist Alice Ludvig (2006, p. 245) argues that it is impossible to take into account all significant differences in the intersectional approach. This one interview was completed over nine and a half hours, several weeks, in four sessions, between February and May 2005. She started with the open question and statement: 'I am interested in your life-story. Please tell me everything that comes to your mind and that you would like to tell' (Ludvig, 2006, p. 250). Ludvig then analysed the woman's 'self-positioning in a specific setting in time and place', to examine their effects on the 'particularities' of gender, class and ethnicity (Ludvig, 2006, p. 251), providing insights into the ways in which one single actor is structurally positioned. This qualitative in-depth process of gathering life narratives enables the exploration of how and what diverse aspects of an individual's life and identity intersect. She then examined this narrative more structurally, by asking the question: 'What does this interview tell us about the politico-social structures in Austria?' (Ludvig, 2006, p. 250). This approach resonates with the qualitative research that I have undertaken in Australia that used narrative interviews to gather diverse perspectives of home and homelessness, including the experiences of service users (Zufferey and Kerr, 2004; Zufferey, 2015).

My research

Since 2001, I have researched home and homelessness in numerous research projects. I have already discussed four of these research projects in Chapter 3 (Zufferey and Rowntree, 2014; Zufferey and Chung, 2015; Zufferey, 2015), including our recent study on gendered violence (Zufferey *et al.*, 2016). In Chapter 5, I presented my research on the perspectives of social workers. This chapter particularly discusses the narratives of people who experienced homelessness (Zufferey and Kerr, 2004), briefly mentions findings from our research on ageing and sexuality (Rowntree and Zufferey, 2015) and further explores my intersectional research on the experiences of home and homelessness (as mentioned in Chapter 3), focusing on refugee, migration and middle-class narratives of home (Zufferey, 2015).

Prior to becoming an academic, I worked as a social work practitioner in different fields of practice and geographical locations. I worked in remote

Western Australia where my client group was primarily Aboriginal families and communities, in London, UK in the fields of aged care and disability, and in Adelaide, South Australia, with people who experienced homelessness and mental illness. This last area of work led to my interest in researching diverse experiences of homelessness. Influenced by sociological ethnographic studies that examined the identity talk of people who experience homelessness (Snow and Anderson, 1987; 1993; Snow *et al.*, 2007), the research I discuss next was my MSW research that gathered nine stories of Aboriginal and non-Aboriginal men and women in Adelaide, South Australia. I found that whilst people have been identified and categorised as being 'homeless' by social workers and policy makers, they often did not identify themselves as 'homeless' (Zufferey and Kerr, 2004). The sample comprised four women and five men, four being of Aboriginal background (three women and one man), four of non-Aboriginal background and one man of European Australian background. Their ages ranged between 23 and 73, and the duration of their homelessness had lasted between six weeks to 20 years. All except for one young woman had experienced 'sleeping rough'. This chapter revisits some of the findings of this study that have also been published elsewhere in different detail (see Zufferey and Kerr, 2004). To contextualise the study, I emphasise literature about the effects of colonisation and then discuss how homelessness affected people's subjectivities.

Colonisation

In Australia, Aboriginal people make up 3 per cent of the Australian population but are over 20 per cent of the homeless population. These statistics point to the need to examine homelessness from the perspectives of Aboriginal people, to develop a multilayered analysis that is inclusive of the historical effects of racism, Indigenous dispossession and colonisation (Briskman, 2003; Green and Baldry, 2008, p. 389). Aboriginal and Torres Strait Islander people are overrepresented in the Australian homelessness statistics, more likely to be sleeping rough, in improvised and overcrowded dwellings and less likely to be homeowners (AIHW, 2011). Aboriginal Australians are the most disadvantaged group in Australia on a wide range of socio-economic indicators such as health, income, education, employment and housing. They are at increasing risk of being defined as 'homeless' and of feeling 'spiritually homeless', in the context of the history of colonisation and their dispossession from their land and 'sense of belonging, home and place' (Keys Young, 1998; Moreton-Robinson, 2003, p. 23; Moreton-Robinson, 2009).

The disempowering effects of colonisation can also be found in other countries such as Canada and the USA. Hulko (2015, p. 85) has gathered the perspectives of First Nation Elders about living with dementia using intersectionality, and argued the importance of co-sharing research findings in ways that 'position members of equity seeking groups as meaning makers and knowledge creators', to influence social change. Globally, post-colonial studies examine the effects of colonising practices that marginalise large groups of people on the basis of ethnicity, gender and class, to name a few (Young, 2003). In my research, the perspectives of colonised peoples from Aboriginal Australian cultural backgrounds are given particular attention. These alternative perspectives can provide social workers with ways to unsettle dominant Westernised assumptions about policy and practice responses to homelessness (Zufferey and Chung, 2015).

In the context of countries that have been colonised, Aboriginal people are disadvantaged by colonial histories and government policies that removed them from their lands, and removed children from their families. Indeed, people were (and still are) 'made homeless' by government policies (Lester, 1999, p. 18). Government policies have been constructed by people in power (such as social workers), with particular privileges, based on their membership of a particular dominant group. Privilege is invisible. The privileged groups have the power to determine social norms, naturalise privilege and the sense of entitlement that accompanies it (Pease, 2010). Social workers have directly participated in these social interventions related to the removal of children and creation of homelessness. I have previously reflected on my involvement in child protection services as an example of how current 'child protection' policies and legislation are biased in favour of white people who have the invisible power and privilege to create policy and legislation that is not always culturally relevant for Aboriginal communities (Walter *et al.*, 2011; Zufferey, 2013).

The effects of 'being stolen' from one's country, land, community and family has disempowering, intergenerational effects on people's lives, increasing the risks of experiencing and feeling 'homeless':

> I just get angry … you got rich from our country, you stole it from us. You stole my family, you stolen me from my family, which in turn has affected my children and my grandchildren. It's not just my children … I've got my grandchildren in foster care … my little ones that are stolen within the system. Just like I was. That's what keeps me going [advocating against the system].
>
> (Aboriginal woman, aged 43)

As Pease (2010, p. 109) argues, 'people's perceptions of the world are influenced by their personal biographies and social location'. This quote refers to Stolen Generation/s policies that occurred in the context of race and class privileges of the dominant colonising group, which relates to 'who decides' and 'who benefits' from policy constructions and decisions (see Zufferey, 2013 for more details). The power dynamics and social injustices of these colonising practices that 'stole' Aboriginal people's land and families is repeated in intergenerational experiences of family members being 'stolen' by the child protection system. These foundational injustices are central to the Australian context of homelessness.

Next, I discuss how diverse experiences and perspectives on homelessness are constituted by resistances to dominant social work practices; complex feelings of being 'degraded', 'unwanted' as well as 'lucky'; advocating for Aboriginal land rights, as well as challenging dichotomous constructions of 'black and white' issues through 'streetie' discourses.

Resistances

Despite feeling disempowered by the responses of service systems, service users can also resist social work practices that 'tell them what to do'. For example, two women of Aboriginal background explained that they would prefer to 'sleep rough' than be 'told what to do' by services:

> I had untold people coming in and saying 'right we are going to do this ... we are going to do that'. I'm sitting there going ... hang on I'm here you know! And then that is when I get up and run away and go and sleep on the streets, cause I found it better out there. At least I had a sense of freedom. No-one was telling me what to do.
>
> (Aboriginal woman, aged 45)

Similarly, 'I would rather stay on the streets than go to a place where I am told when I'm allowed to go out and when I am not' (Aboriginal woman, aged 43).

The quotes above show that these two Aboriginal women do not find current homelessness service approaches respectful or self-determining. They imply that collaborative and strengths-based social work practices would improve engagement with potential service users and more positively respond to people who are 'sleeping rough' (see also Zufferey and Kerr, 2004, p. 350). 'One size fits all' policy responses and practices within services are often influenced by medical and scientific discourses that can construct deficit and homogenous categories to represent people who experience homelessness (Zufferey and Kerr, 2004). An intersectional social work approach, on the other hand, acknowledges the effects of intersecting social injustices and power relations that can contribute to processes of social marginalisation and social exclusion.

Degraded into nothingness

Whilst service users can resist social work interventions in their lives, negative representations of 'homeless people' can, nonetheless, constitute their subjectivities. For example, people who experience homelessness can have an overwhelming feeling that they are being 'put down' or excluded from society, as illustrated in the following two quotes from older men who have experienced homelessness. This can be a feeling of being degraded into 'a nothingness': 'It makes you feel degraded and low and nothingness. I am a nothingness. I am being put down by society. I am useless. I am no good' (non-Aboriginal man, aged 50). In the next quote similar sentiments are described as an 'unwanted complex' with a long history, likely tracing back to childhood experiences: 'You feel unwanted, unloved, no-one wants a drunk do they? ... resenting authority, in and out of jail, locking me up and unwanted, a problem of unwantedness ... a sort of unwanted complex' (non-Aboriginal man, aged 73). These feelings of being unwanted or excluded can then lead to feelings of self-blame for being in a homeless predicament: 'It [homelessness] makes you think what could have been ... no-one else to blame but yourself' (Aboriginal man, aged 50). This sentiment illustrates the effects of negative societal representations and approaches to homelessness that are situated within broader Western individualist, neoliberal discourses about social problems, emphasising individual self-interest and moral responsibility for one's own problems (Harris, 2003; Zufferey and Kerr, 2004; Jamrozik, 2005; Gordon and Zufferey, 2013).

The morally ascribed responsibility for oneself can constitute the subjectivities of people who experience homelessness and are in turn, deployed to describe the subjectivities of 'other' homeless people. This process is evident in a quote by one of the young women who argued that some people are homeless and 'in the shit because they are shit ... no desire to pull themselves out of their situation' (non-Aboriginal woman, aged 23). In contrast, another service user shifted the responsibilities for homelessness from individuals to society: 'Society has admitted they are incompetent; they can't solve this problem of homelessness. They are instigators of homelessness in the first place, the government body, the bureaucrats' (non-Aboriginal man, aged 50). In some circumstances, people blame themselves (and other individuals) for being homeless but in other circumstances, the same individuals may blame society. This contradictory attitude highlights the complexities of diverse perspectives on homelessness, which is conceived as being both an individual and community responsibility (see also Zufferey and Kerr, 2004, pp. 347–348). Expanding on this analysis, an intersectional approach can highlight how social structures, individual subjectivities and discursive representations of social problems can variously shape perspectives and experiences of homelessness.

To emphasise broader concerns about society, policies and social work practice, both Aboriginal and non-Aboriginal advocates drew on the notion of citizenship: 'We are homeless Australian citizens, not scum, not junkies' (non-Aboriginal man, aged 50). In particular, Aboriginal people in Australia were not considered 'citizens' with equal rights and self-determination: 'we weren't citizens of this country. Welfare, or the Department, anyone had the right to walk in and take us away' (recounting the effects of the Stolen Generation/s from an Aboriginal Australian/Indigenous perspective, Lester, 1999, p. 18). As well as being racialised, citizenship is historically, politically and conceptually gendered (Lister, 2003). One woman expressed this as 'being treated as lesser beings': 'That is what it comes down to … God's a man and women are treated as lesser beings … it's all based on a patriarchal God' (recounting the effects of gender from the perspective of a 23-year-old non-Aboriginal woman). Despite these more negative assertions, people who experienced homelessness also felt 'lucky', more knowledgeable about 'the other side of life' or the 'other reality' of homelessness.

I'm lucky …

Two women of different ages and cultural backgrounds expressed their feelings of being 'blessed', 'lucky' and 'stronger' to have experienced homelessness:

> I really respect all the streeties … it's made me stronger … it's made me appreciate little things … I feel blessed that I have been able to experience that life … cause I know that I can't judge, I won't judge, how can I judge?
>
> (Aboriginal woman, aged 43)

This quote illustrated a respect for the collective named as 'streeties'. As evident in the quote below, social workers are also perceived to have knowledge about this 'other side' of life:

> I am lucky actually. I know the other side. I know this side and I am lucky to have that knowledge … I consider myself to have more knowledge on life than these people who have gone to university and got a job … unless they become social workers … they'll never see it … they'll just live their whole life, just walk past people in the street and look down on them.
>
> (non-Aboriginal woman, aged 23)

These standpoints resonate with the findings of Boydell *et al.*'s (2000, p. 8) Canadian study into adult shelter users, who reported that homelessness 'gave them a deeper understanding of life and its meaning'. An intersectional social work approach can contribute to mutually co-constructed meanings and experiences of homelessness, depending on the social contexts and categories of difference being examined by the researcher.

A 'black and white' issue?

When exploring racism, Aboriginal participants did name its oppressive effects. The historical connection to land was emphasised by Aboriginal people who were, at the time of the interviews, being 'moved on' from inner city locations, during the introduction of dry zone legislation in Adelaide, South Australia (see also Zufferey and Kerr, 2004). As one Aboriginal woman said, the land 'it is them': 'Find out whose land you're really running your cars on. Whose land is this underneath all your little cement? This is Kaurna country [belongs to the local Aboriginal people]. It's that mob. It is them'

(Aboriginal woman, aged 43). As well, inner city locations that were being gentrified were historical 'meeting places', as explained by this Aboriginal man: 'If you go up to the city, that's the first place you go to (Victoria Square). It's a meeting place. My tribe the Ngarrindjeri tribe, it was our territory before' (Aboriginal man, aged 50).

However, some Aboriginal and non-Aboriginal women and men resisted dichotomous constructions of 'black and white' issues. When speaking about the 'homeless culture' or connections between people who are homeless ('streeties'), the theme of connection and reciprocity with other 'streeties' was dominant. This attitude related to people who are homeless 'helping each other out', materially and emotionally (Zufferey, 2001; see also Zufferey and Kerr, 2004, p. 348). As one man said:

> I am thinking of others, what their needs are … Everyone goes out with feelers and tries to get it [money, alcohol, cigarettes, drugs, food] for the people, so it is like a network within itself … My day to day routine would be that, communicating with other people who are in the same situation as me, attending and caring for them, them attending and caring for others. It is a chain reaction and we are looking out for our needs.
>
> (non-Aboriginal man, aged 50)

Like this non-Aboriginal man, other older men of Aboriginal cultural background also reported sharing their alcohol and drugs with other 'streeties', in the 'chain reaction' of 'caring for others'.

The Aboriginal woman below stated her opinion that homelessness was not a 'black and white' issue:

> Up town you will find it is not a black and white issue … white people are camping right next to nunga [Aboriginal] people … you get a lot of tribal people come here, to live with them you gotta be fairly tough. If you're a streetie, you're a streetie, it doesn't matter. If someone robs you, well then you've got all the streeties you know. They look out for each other. Some of them don't … some of them like want to just come and go … make their money [e.g. drug dealers].
>
> (Aboriginal woman, aged 45)

Therefore, the feelings of solidarity with other people who experience homelessness ('streeties') can transcend unequal race relations and racial differences. However, not all 'streeties' 'look out for each other'. This Aboriginal woman excludes 'drug dealers' from the 'streetie' collective, who are constructed as being predominantly self-interested.

These identification complexities in the perspectives of people who experience homelessness have also been found by American sociologists Wasserman and Clair (2010). They observed a man they called Carnell, who they labelled as 'intelligent, articulate and clever', trying to convince another man that 'black and white don't exist' (Wasserman and Clair, 2010, p. 17). They observed that 'while he did not have an academic vocabulary, as he talked, it was clear that his thoughts went beyond the I-don't-see-color cliché to a deeply philosophical, social constructionist view of race and ethnicity'. For example, 'What color are you?' his debate partner challenged, ''cause I'm black.' Carnell wouldn't budge, 'There is no black; they made that shit up' (Carnell, in Wasserman and Clair, 2010, p. 17). However, they also noted that this social constructionist position on race relations is unusual.

In a different context, Larry Dillard recounts his experiences on the streets and prison, in Blauner's (1990, p. 111) book, on stories from the civil rights movement in America. He speaks about 'taking sides': 'The brothers stay together and we call that respect. Togetherness. Like, a brother, he don't have no white friends. If he do, you're a dead brother. You're a D.B. White on black, two-tone. You on a side.' The civil rights movement asserted the rights of citizens to political and social freedom and equality and thus, one had to take 'a side' against these racialised (and gendered) injustices. In the context of researching literal homelessness in New York, Passaro (2014) argued that gender, race and family status are culturally embedded moral and social locations that determined chances of exiting homelessness. She found that the persistently homeless 'on the streets' are overwhelmingly black men who tend to be excluded from the service system (Passaro, 2014). In contrast, women's experiences of homelessness are often less visible than men's because they are more likely to experience living in temporary shelters, 'couch (or sofa in the UK) surfing' or staying with friends and family (Murray, 2011). However, there are some women who also 'sleep rough' and live 'on the streets' but this homeless circumstance poses high risks to their safety.

Women's homelessness

For women who do 'sleep rough', they tend to engage in strategies that render them invisible. Sociologists in the UK, Casey *et al.* (2008), gathered data from a questionnaire survey of 144 single homeless women without children and 44 interviews with women in Leeds, London, Sheffield and Norwich, England who did use public spaces as their 'home' (Casey *et al.*, 2008, p. 913). The sample included women who had stayed temporarily in hostels, bed and breakfast hotels, refuges, squats, with friends and family, with strangers and on the streets (Casey *et al.*, 2008, p. 901). Aged between 16 and 59 years old, 30 per cent were from minority ethnic groups, of African Caribbean, Black African, British Asian, Irish, Roma Gypsy and 'Other White' origin. The women who experienced homelessness did occupy public spaces, such as public toilets, museums, art galleries, libraries, hospitals, airports, car parks and 'the space surrounding public and private buildings' (Casey *et al.*, 2008, p. 903). The study found that women 'actively and strategically use these spaces to their own ends, and for their own needs and purposes, extracting and deriving positive benefit from them' (Casey *et al.*, 2008, p. 905). They resisted the rules of public spaces by 'engaging in identity work' by not being labelled as 'homeless' (Casey *et al.*, 2008, p. 899). These strategies included: presenting as 'respectable', avoiding 'well-known places on the streets' where groups of homeless people congregate and sleep, avoiding being detected by timekeeping their use of space, developing relationships with gatekeepers (such as security guards or toilet attendants) and 'projecting an image of toughness', to avoid 'unwelcome advances of other homeless people', as well as workers from homeless agencies intent on 'rescuing them' (Casey *et al.*, 2008, pp. 909–911). The employment of these strategies assisted the women to negotiate the practical, emotional and ontological impacts of literal homelessness (Casey *et al.*, 2008, p. 901). Women experience homelessness differently to men and this also depends on their social and geographical locations, including urban-rural contexts.

The main cause of women's homelessness is domestic and family violence, which has gendered and racialised aspects. In Australia, Indigenous women experience up to 38 times the rate of hospitalisation compared to other females, for spouse/domestic partner-inflicted assaults (Al-Yaman *et al.*, 2006). American Indigenous feminist author Andrea Smith (2005) argues that violence against women cannot be separated from the violence of the State, from patriarchy, colonialism and white supremacy. That is, that Indigenous sovereignty and sexual violence cannot be separated because the appropriation of Indigenous land occurred (and still occurs) through gendered violence. In my small Australian study, the Aboriginal women who experienced literal homelessness discussed both racial discrimination as well as unequal gendered relations. In regard to gendered violence, the Aboriginal woman below expressed the feeling of 'not being safe' as a woman when 'sleeping rough', being obligated to 'have a partner' or 'a group' for protection and choosing the 'wrong' violent man:

> You more or less have to have a partner. Or you've got to stick with a group ... to keep you warm and look after you ... but it doesn't always work ... some partners, chosen the wrong ones, turn out to be the most violent of the lot ... I've slept by myself ... but you don't sleep ... you just lay there.
>
> (Aboriginal woman, aged 43)

As evident in this quote, while women experience homelessness because of domestic and family violence, they are also likely to experience further violence while homeless (Murray, 2011).

As well, in Australia, young women have the highest rate of assistance by homeless services. Watson's (2011, p. 639) study of 15 young women in Australia about 'survival sex' positioned its occurrence within a context of gendered discourses. She found that the young women held a sense of personal responsibility for managing their own situations. She concluded that young women experiencing homelessness are 'subject to the pressures of individualisation that have been produced by the neoliberal policies of Western capitalist societies', in which they 'are required to find individual solutions to structural problems' (Watson, 2011, p. 639). These social inequalities reinforce community attitudes and social norms that support violence against women, leaving many unjust gendered (and racialised) practices unquestioned (Pease and Flood, 2008, p. 547; Zufferey *et al.*, 2016).

Sexuality

When exploring gender and sexuality, the literature on sexuality and homelessness is sparse. Sexuality has received less attention than other axes of social analysis in the fields of social work (Rowntree, 2014) and homelessness (Zufferey and Rowntree, 2014). One out of the nine stories of homelessness that I draw on in this chapter spoke of the effects of heterosexual dominance (Zufferey and Kerr, 2004). Heteronormativity is how 'heterosexual privilege is woven into the fabric of social life, pervasively and insidiously, ordering everyday existence' (Jackson, 2006, p. 108). One young non-Aboriginal woman claimed that homophobia in 'the homeless situation, it's even worse than normal society' and expressed how she felt empowered when marching in the Pride March: 'I marched in the Pride March ... I realised the meaning of pride ... it's not just about being gay ... it's saying ... pride ... and gay or straight ... don't pick on me ... I'm not going to take it!' (non-Aboriginal woman, aged 23). This young woman is clearly voicing resistance to dominant heterosexual norms from a social justice and human rights advocacy perspective: 'don't pick on me ... I'm not going to take it!'

Previous research has found that homophobia in the family home (and the wider society) increases young people's risk of experiencing homelessness (Dunne *et al.*, 2002). Social discrimination related to sexual identity can contribute to the loss of 'home' and the onset of homelessness (Gold, 2005). The heterosexual, nuclear family home is held up as the 'emblematic model of comfort, care and belonging' (Ahmed *et al.*, 2003; Fortier, 2003, p. 115). However, young people often flee unsupportive family homes in the process of 'coming out' to more freely express their sexual identities in adulthood (Pilkey, 2013a; 2013b). In contrast to the idea of the nuclear family home as being essentially homophobic, Australian social geographer Andrew Gorman Murray (2008, p. 31) considers the experience of GLB youth who are well-supported by parents and siblings. He argues that family homes can become sites of resistance to wider practices of heterosexism, and that heterosexual identity does not 'essentially' generate heterosexist reactions and attitudes, but can make space for non-heterosexual subjectivities (Gorman Murray, 2008, p. 31). When considering an intersectional social work approach to homelessness, the complicated relationships between sexuality, age, homophobia and experiences of home cannot be ignored.

As well, Gorman Murray (2007, p. 229) explored the meanings of home for middle-class gay men and lesbians living in urban Australia using data from 37 in-depth interviews. He noted that normative meanings of home relate to privacy, identity and being with family but that they also vary across social groups, according to gender, race, class, age, disability and sexuality. He argues that meanings of home are being reinterpreted by gays and lesbians, and that their experiences in contemporary society can generate 'homes that affirm sexual difference' (Gorman Murray, 2007, p. 229). In our smaller study on the lived and imagined experiences of home and sexuality, the perspectives of men and women differed (Zufferey and Rowntree, 2014). Using data from a focus group of six women and individual interviews with three women, all who identified as lesbian, the women tended to construct home and community as belonging to a collective based on sexual orientation (Zufferey and Rowntree, 2014). In contrast, the two men interviewed who identified as gay or bisexual did not identify strongly with a sexuality-based collective as 'home'.

Ageing and sexuality

When intersecting age and sexuality, the sexual expression of older people is an emerging area of study, although not specifically in homelessness. This literature tends to focus on the responses of staff in aged care settings to older people's sexual expression (Petriwskyj *et al.*, 2015), which is inextricably linked to residents feeling a sense of belonging and connection to being at 'home' within these facilities. In our Australian study that explored the expression of sexual intimacy in aged care settings, the perspectives of staff differed from community members (Rowntree and Zufferey, 2015). We found that staff members were more drawn to ideas underpinning a 'needs' discourse, informing residential aged care policies, procedures and practices that authorise and give power to staff, to meet residents' sexual 'needs'. On the other hand, community members favoured ideas that are consistent with a 'rights' discourse that aim to improve residents' privacy and autonomy, by shifting the balance of power towards them (Rowntree and Zufferey, 2015). The total sample in our focus groups and individual interviews comprised 42 participants, of which 19 were staff members (18 women and 1 man) and 23 community members (15 women and 8 men), ranged in age from 24 to 86 years and of diverse cultural backgrounds (seven staff members were born overseas). One community member, who was also an aged care resident expressed indignation about the erosion of her rights, autonomy and privacy in her life since moving into aged care, which she did not consider assisted her to feel 'at home'. For example, while being assisted with her shower, a nurse announced that the doctor was there to see her and asked if he could come in. She said:

Certainly not, either they can come back later or I'll see them next week. I was highly incensed... . You're always telling me this is my home. If I were at home, there would be no way that I would entertain a doctor while I was in the shower.

(86 year-old heterosexual widow, retired nurse)

Our research highlighted clear power differences between service providers, residents and community members and this related to how they viewed older people's sexual expression (see also Rowntree and Zufferey, 2015). In the context of ageist social structures and institutions, older people are potentially subjected to oppressive social practices related to intersecting markers of age, gender and sexuality, that affect their sense of belonging and how 'at home' they feel in aged care facilities (and in society more broadly).

Furthermore, research indicates that older women who live alone are at greater risk of homelessness because they 'will be poorer than men their age, less able to maintain homeownership, and less able to compete in the private rental market for affordable accommodation' (McFerran, 2010, p. 79). Disadvantaging gendered social locations are evident in 'the entrenched social and economic disadvantage that continues to separate the experiences of women and men', and which intersects class, gender and age (McFerran, 2010, p. 79). Age can intersect with other areas of potential disadvantage such as ability, sexuality, gender, ethnicity and socioeconomic inequalities that contribute to increasing the risks of homelessness. Another aspect of age relates to children and homelessness.

The voices of children

In regard to children, there is a considerable amount of literature that focuses on the negative effects of homelessness on their physical and mental health, education, community and social connections, behaviour, emotions (such as grief and loss) and potential future aspirations (Buckner, 2008; Kirkman *et al.*, 2009; Gibson and Morphett, 2011). Family and children's homelessness occurs in the contexts of domestic and family violence, mental illness, substance abuse, poverty, child abuse and lack of housing affordability and suitability. Parents coping with homelessness and multiple stressors do acknowledge that their capacity to address their children's needs is temporarily impaired (Gibson and Morphett, 2011, p. 23).Varney and van Vliet (2008) argued that supportive housing programmes and interventions need to be tailored to children and address multiple needs. The use of child centred approaches to respond to children who are homeless would involve: engaging them through play, reassuring them that they are not alone or to blame, showing genuine respect, working according to children's developmental capabilities and asking them their understandings of events (Thomas, 2007; Gibson and Morphett, 2011). However, children's experiences are likely to differ according to their abilities, social locations, gender and cultural backgrounds. Drawing on intersectional feminism, Damant *et al.* (2008, p. 123) argue that intersectional feminism is a promising approach to 'explore the multiple and complex links among domestic violence, child abuse, and mothering' and relevant 'social identities and systems of oppression'.

The diverse voices of children who are homeless are important to hear (Mustafa, 2004; Moore *et al.*, 2008). Children who are homeless can experience loss, shame, ostracism and labelling (Anooshian, 2003). Similarly to other countries, in the UK, black and minority ethnic children are also over-represented among homeless households (Mustafa, 2004). A report called 'Listen Up' by Zoya Mustafa (2004, p. 6) for Shelter UK gathered the voices of 29 (17 boys and 12 girls) children aged between 4 and 16, from a wide range of nationalities and ethnicities, documenting their views, thoughts and feelings about experiencing homelessness. The method used to collect data from the children were writing and drawing in activity books, completing a questionnaire and participating in drama exercises (Mustafa, 2004, p. 6), depending on age. The themes discussed by children about their everyday experiences of homelessness included: housing conditions, health and well-being, schools and education, leisure and play, unsafe local environments, broken relationships and the emotional effects of homelessness (Mustafa, 2004). Experiences of homelessness are considerably disruptive to children:

> for four months we didn't go to school, we went to six houses, no, seven houses and six new schools ... I don't like moving, because every time I make new friends and then I have to move again and again and again.
>
> (Girl, 10, in Mustafa, 2004, p. 9)

In addition to being homeless in London, many of the children in the study from 11 different ethnic groups, had to deal with cultural and language barriers. Adverse experiences early in life for children of diverse backgrounds can have negative impacts (Perry, 2002) that then intersect with other social discriminations, based on nationality, race, ethnicity, class, gender and sex (to name a few). In the above UK study, culturally diverse children commonly felt socially isolated because of limited school attendance, and living in cramped and unsuitable accommodation. They also expressed feeling anxious about 'what was acceptable within British culture' (Mustafa, 2004, p. 27). An intersectional approach would enable social workers to be aware of shifting exclusionary discourses, to critically examine systemic inequalities and institutionalised classism, sexism and racism, including the intersection of xenoracist discourses with other social inequalities (Masocha and Simpson, 2011).

One female child described the effects of feeling 'othered' because she was living in hotel accommodation 'occupied almost exclusively by other non-British households', and feeling stigmatised due to exclusion from what she considers to be 'English people' (Mustafa, 2004, p. 27). She expressed feeling different from the wider 'English' community due to her housing situation:

There are lots of Arabs in the hotel ... lots of Arabs with children and lots of Chinese. I didn't see much English people but it's full of Chinese and Arab people ... I'd like to see some English people because it's their place anyway, that's the only English person I've seen so far is the security, the three security men.

(Girl, 10, in Mustafa, 2004, p. 27)

Thinking about these intersectional disadvantages facing children who are homeless enables social workers to respond better to these diverse experiences and unequal social relations that constitute homelessness.

There is considerable evidence that young people aging out of foster care are at high risk of homelessness (Dworsky and Courtney, 2009). In the USA, in 2009–2010, 59 per cent of children in the foster care system were 'children of color' and 22 per cent became homeless after aging out of the foster care system, compared to 2.6 per cent of the general population of 18–24 year olds, in that given year (AFCARS, 2009). In 2014, this trend continued, with African American and Hispanic children accounting for 24 per cent and 22 per cent, respectively, of children in foster care (AFCARS, 2014). Similarly, in Australia, structural and racial inequalities, such as the legacy of colonisation, Stolen Generation/s, high levels of poverty, ill health and inadequate housing, contribute to the over-representation of Aboriginal children in the child protection system. These children are up to seven times more likely to experience child maltreatment (primarily neglect, physical abuse and emotional abuse) compared to non-Indigenous children (Hunter, 2008). These statistics illustrate the importance of social workers responding to children's homelessness from an intersectional approach, which would include intersecting socio-economic dis/advantages, gendered and racialised inequalities. Furthermore, an understanding of 'adultism' and adult privilege would assist social workers to finds ways of co-designing research and creatively engaging with children, so their voices can be made more visible in homelessness research and practice (Pease, 2010).

Intersections in youth homelessness

Youth homelessness is also a highly researched topic. Hickler and Auerswald (2009) explored the 'worlds' of white and black youth (aged 15–24) who were perceived to be homeless in San Francisco, through gender and ethnicity. They highlighted differences and similarities in pathways to homelessness, self-perceptions, survival strategies and the health of African American and white homeless youth. They initially engaged in participant observation and conducted ethnographic interviews with 54 young people (29 females and 25 males; 25 white, 2 Latino, and 27 African American), of whom 49 were street-recruited and 5 programme-recruited (Hickler and Auerswald, 2009, p. 825). The findings were then validated using concurrent epidemiological data collected from a sample of 205 youth, included 132 male, 66 female and 7 transgender participants, of whom 171 were street-recruited and 34 programme-recruited (Hickler and Auerswald, 2009 p. 826). They found that both ethnic groups shared common childhood histories but that white youth generally identified with the term 'homeless' and engaged in survival activities associated with accessed youth homeless services. In contrast, the sample of African American youth generally did not see themselves as 'homeless', possibly because of the stigma attached to the term, and therefore, 'they were less likely to utilize, or be accessed by, relevant services' (Hickler and Auerswald, 2009, p. 824). This reluctance by the young African American people to identify as 'homeless' and access services could be related to not knowing what services exist or patronising responses they may have received from services. Unlike Australian author Watson (2011) who researched the survival sex (trading sex for food, a place to sleep, other basic needs or drugs) of young women *only*, this study found that overall, 16 per cent of the young people (both male and female) reported that they engaged in 'survival sex', which did not differ by race or gender (Hickler and Auerswald, 2009, p. 828). This has further disempowering ramifications for young people, their experiences of homelessness and subjectivities.

Young people who are defined as 'homeless' but do not identify as being homeless are potentially influenced by simplistic and negative media coverage of homelessness that depicts negative representations (Hodgetts *et al.*, 2006, p. 498). In London, Hodgetts *et al.*'s (2006, p. 497) study found that whilst homeless people emphasised aspects of their lives not present in media portrayals, they also represented themselves 'through common media storylines', invoking a normalising discourse. Hodgetts *et al.* (2006, p. 499) concluded that 'groups who are marginalised cannot simply locate themselves within their own discourses', for they too are social actors within a particular socio-cultural context, and within intersecting power relations. Therefore, discursive representations of homelessness potentially have material effects, which contribute to young people being less likely to access services.

To examine the intersections of youth, race, masculinity and place, Canadian geographer May (2014) conducted 40 interviews and eight 'where-I-live-tours' of the city, with 'Canadian-born young men of colour' (aged 17–26), who have experienced homelessness in the Greater Toronto Area (May, 2014; 2015). He found that race contributes to continuing oppressions based on the intersections of racialised masculinities and homelessness. He notes that suburban areas 'vibrate' a racial 'vibe', compared with the whiteness of downtown Toronto spaces (May, 2015). He concluded that 'racialised and affective landscapes shape, and are shaped by, the masculine performances of the homeless young men of colour in different city spaces' (May, 2014; O'Neill Gutierrez and Hopkins, 2014, p. 3). Following this space-and-place literature in the field of geography that draws on intersectionality, I suggest that social workers can use a similar approach to better understand and theorise youth homelessness.

Narratives of home

Homelessness can be a material reality, as evident in experiences of sleeping rough discussed earlier in this chapter (Zufferey and Kerr, 2004). However, it is also an emotion, a feeling or sense of loss when migrating to a new country or being forced to leave one's 'home country'. As discussed in Chapter 3, to explore narratives of home and homelessness in Adelaide, South Australia, with my colleague Dr Tammy Hand, we conducted 13 semi-structured in-depth interviews about 'home' with three men and ten women, from different cultural, class and age backgrounds (see Zufferey, 2015, p. 15). We found three distinct narratives of home: refugee and forced displacement narratives, family migration and mobility narratives and middle-class narratives of home.

For some people who have migrated, their new country is still becoming home, due to feelings of cultural displacement (Ahmed *et al.*, 2003). In our Australian study, refugees and migrants who have had to flee an unsafe country (and 'home') to a new country and culture experienced feeling disconnected and grieved for their families. For example, a 21-year-old young man on a humanitarian visa said:

> I'm living here, my home is here [in Australia] … In Afghanistan, I didn't, did a good life, because I lost my father, I lost my mother, I lost my life, I couldn't go to school … I think my home is now here, I'm safe … I'm so happy, they accept me to come to Australia.

Despite connecting with Australia as 'home', this young man felt very 'alone' and 'sad' without his family members, and at times felt 'hopeless'. Yet, he did not identify as feeling or being 'homeless' because he was living in a house. In contrast, a 21-year-old woman who was a refugee on a Woman at Risk visa stated feeling 'homeless' in Australia because she was not feeling 'mentally or physically comfortable … right now in my situation, mentally we can say I'm homeless'. These narratives showed emotional connections to 'home' as family and country. However, this young woman's sense of not belonging intersected with her physical and emotional wellbeing, which can contribute to feeling 'homeless', even when living in a house, in a new, safer country. These two refugee narratives indicated that subjective understandings of homelessness differ and may intersect with other experiences such as loss of family, gendered violence and mental and physical health.

Seven of the 13 narratives in this study of home were from people who had recently (voluntarily) migrated to Australia or had memories of family migration. Migration narratives also reflected diverse subjective experiences of home, which included 'being at home' (asking questions such as: Am I or am I not 'at home' in Australia?), 'leaving home' (Should I have left my country?) and 'going home' (Where is home now?) (Ahmed *et al.*, 2003). For example, a 27-year-old married woman of South American background expressed difficulties in transitioning to, and 'feeling at home', in Australia. Instead, she stated 'feeling homeless' without her extended family. Similar to the two young people of refugees backgrounds, her meanings of home and feelings of belonging related to connections with supportive family and friends, who lived elsewhere.

Family migration narratives had a consistent theme about travel and mobility in the past, present and imagined future, mostly unconnected to a physical locality (Ahmed *et al.*, 2003). For example, one 29-year-old woman of mixed cultural background, including Aboriginal Australian origin, constantly moved during her childhood with her parents who were missionaries. Affecting her current connection to home, she described herself as: 'pretty transient ... I find it really hard to settle. I find it really hard to stay somewhere for any amount of time'. Yet, she does not identify as 'homeless', explaining that: 'there's many people travelling the world who live in backpackers and they are not homeless people'. As well, she said, even when 'sleeping rough', Aboriginal people are living 'at home' on their land and 'country': 'they are on their land and they're home'. This view resonates with my earlier studies about Aboriginal Australian connections to land as home and spiritual notions of homelessness, such as when people were removed from their land, communities and families (Zufferey and Kerr, 2004).

Middle-class narratives of home were evident in the stories of three women (two aged in their thirties and one in her fifties) and one man (aged in his thirties), who had no recent experience of family migration and were mostly of Caucasian origin. They were all homeowners and had never felt 'homeless'. These narratives tended to focus on 'home' as owning and renovating a 'house' (or a number of houses), which symbolised financial security and the 'production of middle class identities' (Dowling and Power, 2012, p. 605). These narratives reflect meanings of home as a house, including a sense of financial security, stability, privacy, safety and the ability to control a living space, such as through house renovations and extensions (Gurney, 1999). For example, one 36-year-old married man bought his first house at 23 years of age and paid it off by the time he was 30. He said: 'I've never lived in a rented house'. Now that he and his wife have a child, they are concerned about the 'school zone' and socio-economic location of their house, and are considering moving. His 'ideal' home is: 'if money grew on trees, I'd have another beach side home in an even more glamorous beach suburb'. This homeownership aspiration 'next to the beach' is common in Australia. Three of these four participants (all in their 30s) owned investment properties. One 32-year-old married woman, with aspirations to have children in the future, said that they strived to be 'budding capitalists with good investments ... already starting to plan for being self-funded retirees ... have a couple of businesses' and a number of houses. However, what is left invisible in the promotion of multiple homeownership is how owning multiple homes in Australia as an investment and tax incentive has contributed to increasing housing costs, reducing access to affordable housing and increasing homelessness, which affects people who experience intersecting socioeconomic disadvantages disproportionately. The findings of this study are further discussed in Zufferey (2015). I conclude this chapter by promoting participatory and collaborative research designs as a way forward, when researching homelessness from an intersectional social work approach.

Service user-led research

Returning to Housing First policy responses to address chronic homelessness as discussed in Chapter 4, Housing First has aimed to change the 'balance of power between service providers and service users' (Benjaminsen, 2014, p. 12) often found in institutional settings, such as large inner city homeless shelters. This shifting emphasis is evident in service user-led research reported in *Intersectionalities: The Global Journal of Social Work Analysis, Research, Polity and Practice*. One article by Canadian service users Coltman *et al.* (2015) reported on research that explored Housing First, community integration, mental health and homelessness. The study involved a secondary analysis of 14 purposively sampled transcripts from 18-month follow-up interviews in the At Home/Chez Soi Toronto evaluation. It explored how the participants discussed and 'experienced community integration in their day-to-day lives' (Coltman *et al.*, 2015, p. 39). The researchers found that policies, practices and literature on 'community integration' are mainly concerned with external indicators, such as maintaining housing, accessing employment, education, engaging in community activities or improving living skills. Their findings are consistent with literature that indicates that the subjective experiences of communities are neglected, whether they are geographical or based on shared experiences and identities, such as volunteering, social interests and connection to pets (Coltman *et al.*, 2015, p. 46). People also engage with communities on the basis of shared identities related to, for example, sexuality, cultural backgrounds or gender. The authors of this Canadian study advocate for 'helping professionals to focus on ways in which empowerment can be supported', and the importance of relationships in the process of community integration (Coltman *et al.*, 2015, p. 49). They argued for more research on the effects that 'larger systems and policies have on the lives of people who experience mental (ill) health and homelessness' (Coltman *et al.*, 2015, p. 49).

In relation to the impact of housing, they found that it 'was more than just a place to live ... [it provided] safety, security, and a place to get away' (Coltman *et al.*, 2015, p. 47). For example, their participant eight stated:

> It's not just a house for me or an apartment, it's a home and I love it there. I love the security it gives me. You know, sense of security and sense of, now this is my own apartment as long as I pay the rent.
>
> (in Coltman *et al.*, 2015, p. 47)

Housing provided people with a feeling of 'home', security and self-worth. Housing symbolised that they were functioning members of society, connected to the geographical neighbourhood and to the people in surrounding living units.

Some participants, however, noted that they were happy with their housing but not their neighbourhood, which related to violence and drugs (Coltman *et al.*, 2015). In some instances, hate crimes had a direct impact on people's safety, including discriminatory homophobic attacks, as evident in derogatory language written on the doors of their housing, based on their presumed sexual orientation. Participant one shared: 'Uh, yeah, yeah that's why I'm, another reason I am moving so, yeah my, I've had uh, fag written over my door, on my windows' (Coltman *et al.*, 2015, p. 48). This quote makes visible the 'hate crimes' that people are subjected to in the context of oppressive homophobic community attitudes and heteronormative practices, which intersects with other areas of oppression in the lives of people who have experienced homelessness.

Overall, this consumer-led study found that experiences of past trauma, substance use, legal issues, disability, food and money insecurity were recurrent themes in service user perspectives on the Housing First approaches (Coltman *et al.*, 2015). On the other hand, themes of self-determination, independence, empowerment, integration and inclusion also emerged in the narratives of people who experience homelessness and mental health problems (Coltman *et al.*, 2015, p. 49). Led by researchers who form part of a Lived Experience Caucus, the study provides an example of service user-led methods and how unequal power relations in the research process can be re-configured. Likewise, I suggest the value of including service user-led methods, alongside 'personal-is-political ethical reflexivity' practices (Chapman *et al.*, 2013, p. 24) in social workers' intersectional approaches to homelessness.

Conclusion

Intersectional social work approaches involve embracing and examining the complexities of social work and homelessness, within a matrix of intersecting social differences, focusing on both privilege and disadvantage. I have assumed that social problems such as homelessness are socially constructed, and these constructions can influence how people come to view themselves (Hodgetts *et al.*, 2006). However, exploring the perspectives of people who experience homelessness confirms that resistances are possible and intersectional oppressions are diverse and not static. Intersectional social work approaches can incorporate shifting and changing experiences of home and homelessness, depending on geographical and social contexts, providing for more diverse understandings of both oppression and privilege (Murphy *et al.*, 2009). Such an approach does not provide definite answers to the research, policy and practice tensions in social work and homelessness. However, the approach does enable the asking of reflexive and inclusive questions about how power intersects in the lived experiences of the homeless, as well as in social work responses to homelessness. As social workers, what do we represent as being favourable or unfavourable intersecting 'social location/s', from whose perspective, why, when and in what context? From the perspectives of people affected by the dominant discourses that construct 'disadvantaged' identity categories, when are intersecting oppressions at the centre of that experience (Murphy *et al.*, 2009, p. 55)? As well, when do social workers need to focus on intersecting privileges as central to their own practices and reflections (Hulko, 2015, p. 72)? These are perpetual reflexive questions for the social work profession.

References

Adoption and Foster Care Reporting System (AFCARS). (2009; 2014). U.S. Department of Health and Human Services, Administration for Children and Families, Administration on Children, Youth and Families, Children's Bureau. Accessed 11 May 2016. www.acf.hhs.gov/programs/cb/research-data-technology/statistics-research/afcars.

Ahmed, S., Castaneda, C., Fortier, A. and Sheller, M. (2003). *Uprootings/regroundings: Questions of home and migration*. Oxford, UK: Berg.

Al-Yaman, F., Van Doeland, M. and Wallis, M. (2006). *Family violence among Aboriginal and Torres Strait Islander peoples*. Cat. no. AIHW 17. Canberra, ACT: AIHW.

Anooshian, L.J. (2003). Social isolation and rejection of homeless children. *Journal of Children and Poverty*, 9(2), 115–134.

Australian Institute of Health and Welfare (AIHW). (2011). *Housing and homelessness services: Access for Aboriginal and Torres Strait Islander people*. Cat. no. HOU 237. Canberra, ACT: AIHW.

Bacchi, C. (2009). *Analysing policy: What's the problem represented to be?* Sydney: Pearson.

Benjaminsen, L. (2014). 'Mindshift' and social work methods in a large-scale Housing First programme in Denmark. (pp. 12–13). In *FEANTSA Magazine: Social work in services with homeless people in a changing European social and political context*. Brussels: European Federation of National Organisations working with the Homeless (AISBL).

Blasi, G.L. (1990). Social policy and social science research on homelessness. *Journal of Social Issues*, 46, 207–219.

Blauner, B. (1990). *Black lives white lives: Three decades of race relations in America*. Berkeley, CA: University of California Press.

Boydell, K., Goering, P. and Morrell-Bellai, T.L. (2000). Narratives of identity: Representation of self in people who are homeless. *Qualitative Health Research*, 10(1), 26–39.

Briskman, L. (2003). Indigenous Australians: Towards postcolonial social work. (pp. 92–106). In J. Allan, B. Pease, and L. Briskman (Eds). *Critical social work*. Crows Nest, NSW: Allen and Unwin.

Buckner, J.C. (2008). Understanding the impact of homelessness on children: Challenges and future directions. *American Behavioral Scientist*, 51(6),721–736.

Casey, R., Goudie, R. and Reeve, K. (2008). Homeless women in public spaces: Strategies of resistance. *Housing Studies*, 23(6), 899–916.

Chapman, C., Hoque, N. and Utting, L. (2013). Fostering a personal-is-political ethics: Reflexive conversations in social work education. *Intersectionalities: A Global Journal of Social Work Analysis, Research, Polity, and Practice*, 2(1), 24–50.

Coltman, L., Gapka, S., Harriott, D., Koo, M., Reid, J. and Zsager, A. (2015). Understanding community integration in a Housing First approach: Toronto at Home/Chez Soi community based research. *Intersectionalities: A Global Journal of Social Work Analysis, Research, Polity and Practice*, 4(2), 39–50.

Damant, D., Lapierre, S., Kouraga, A., Fortin, A., Hamelin-Brabant, L., Lavergne, C. and Lessard, G. (2008). Taking child abuse and mothering into account: Intersectional feminism as an alternative for the study of domestic violence. *Affilia: Journal of Women and Social Work*, 23, 123–133

Dowling, R. and Power, E. (2012). Sizing home: Doing family in Sydney, Australia. *Housing Studies*, 27, 605–619.

Dunne, G.A., Prendergast S. and Telford, D. (2002). Young, gay, homeless and invisible: A growing population? *Culture, Health and Sexuality*, 4, 103–115.

Dworsky, A. and Courtney, M. (2009). Homelessness and the transition from foster care to adulthood among 19 year old former foster youth. *Child Welfare*, 88(4), 23–56.

Fitzpatrick, S. and Christian, J. (2006). Comparing homelessness research in the US and Britain. *International Journal of Housing Policy*, 6(3), 313–333.

Fortier, A. (2003). Making home: Queer migrations and motions of attachment. (pp. 115–135). In S. Ahmed, C. Castaneda, A. Fortier and M. Sheller (2003). *Uprootings/Regroundings: Questions of home and migration*. Oxford, UK: Berg.

Gibson, C. and Morphett, K. (2011). Creative responses to the needs of children: Promising practice. *Developing Practice*, 28, 23–31.

Gold, D. (2005). *Sexual exclusion: Issues and best practice in lesbian, gay and bisexual housing and homelessness*. London: Shelter and Stonewall Housing.

Gordon, L. and Zufferey, C. (2013). Working with diversity in a neoliberal environment. *Advances in Social Work and Welfare Education*, 15(1), 20–30.

Gorman Murray, A. (2007). Reconfiguring domestic values: Meanings of home for gay men and lesbians. *Housing, Theory and Society*, 24(3), 229–246.

Gorman Murray, A. (2008). Queering the family home: Narratives from gay, lesbian and bisexual youth coming out in supportive family homes in Australia. *Gender, Place and Culture: A Journal of Feminist Geography*, 15(1), 31–44.

Green, S. and Baldry, E. (2008). Building Indigenous Australian social work. *Australian Social Work*, 61(4), 389–402.

Gurney, C. (1999). Pride and prejudice: Discourses of normalization in public and private accounts of home ownership. *Housing Studies*, 14, 63–83.

Harris, J. (2003). *The social work business*. London: Routledge.

Hickler, B. and Auerswald, C.L. (2009). The worlds of homeless white and African American youth in San Francisco, California: A cultural epidemiological comparison. *Social Science and Medicine*, 68, 824–831.

Hodgetts, D., Hodgetts, A. and Radley, A. (2006). Life in the shadow of the media: Imaging street homelessness in London. *European Journal of Cultural Studies*, 9, 497–516.

Hulko, W. (2015). Operationalizing intersectionality in feminist social work research: Reflections and techniques from research with equity-seeking groups. (pp. 69–89). In S. Wahab, B. Anderson-Nathe and C. Gringeri (Eds). *Feminisms in social work research*. New York, NY: Routledge.

Hunter, S. (2008). Child maltreatment in remote Aboriginal communities and the Northern Territory Emergency Response: A complex issue. *Australian Social Work*, 61(4), 372–388.

Jackson, S. (2006). Interchanges: Gender, sexuality and heterosexuality: The complexity (and limits) of heteronormativity. *Feminist Theory*, 7(1), 105–121.

Jacobs, K., Kemeny, J. and Manzi, T. (1999). The struggle to define homelessness: A constructivist approach. (pp. 11–28). In S. Hutson and D. Clapham (Eds). *Homelessness: Public policies and private troubles*. London: Cassell.

Jamrozik, A. (2005). *Social policy in the post welfare state*. Melbourne, Vic: Pearson Education.

Keys Young (1998). *Homelessness in the Aboriginal and Torres Strait Islander context and its possible implications for the Supported Accommodation Assistance Program (SAAP)*. Sydney: FaCS.

Kirkman, M., Keys, D., Turner, A. and Bodzak, D. (2009). *'Does camping count?' Children's experiences of homelessness*. Melbourne, Vic: The Salvation Army Australia Southern Territory.

Lester, J. (1999). History and home: An Indigenous Australian perspective, homelessness. Dulwich Centre Publications, Adelaide. *Dulwich Centre Journal*, 3, 18–19.

Lister, R. (2003). *Citizenship: Feminist perspectives*. Basingstoke, UK: Palgrave Macmillan.

Ludvig, A. (2006). Differences between women? Intersecting voices in a female narrative. *European Journal of Women's Studies*, 13(3), 245–258.

McFerran, L. (2010). It could be you: Female, single, older and homeless. *Parity*, 23(10), 15–18.

Masocha, S. and Simpson, M.K. (2011). *Xenoracism: Towards a critical understanding of the construction of asylum seekers and its implications for social work practice*. *Practice: Social Work in Action*, 23(1), 5–18.

May, J. (2014). 'My place of residence': Home and homelessness in the Greater Toronto Area. (pp. 173–187). In M. Gorman Murray and P. Hopkins (Eds). *Masculinities and place*. Aldershot: Ashgate.

May, J. (2015). Racial vibrations, masculine performances: Experiences of homelessness among young men of colour in the Greater Toronto Area. *Gender, Place and Culture: A Journal of Feminist Geography*, 22(3), 405–420.

Moore, T., McArthur, M. and Noble-Carr, D. (2008). 'Stuff you'd never think of': Children talk about homelessness and how they'd like to be supported. *Family Matters*, 78, 36–43.

Moreton-Robinson, A. (2003). I still call Australia home: Indigenous belonging and place in a white postcolonizing society. (pp. 23–40). In S. Ahmed, C. Castaneda, A. Fortier and M. Sheller (Eds). *Uprootings/regroundings: Questions of home and migration*. Oxford UK: Berg.

Moreton-Robinson, A. (2009). *Talkin' up to the white woman*. St Lucia, QLD: University of Queensland Press.

Murphy, Y., Hunt V., Zajicek, A.M., Norris, A.N. and Hamilton, L. (2009). *Incorporating intersectionality in social work practice, research, policy, and education*. Washington, DC: National Association of Social Workers (NASW) Press.

Murray, S. (2011). Violence against homeless women: Safety and social policy. *Australian Social Work*, 64(3), 346–361.

Mustafa, Z. (2004). *Listen up: The voices of homeless children*. London: Shelter.

O'Neill Gutierrez, C. and Hopkins, P. (2014). Introduction: Young people, gender and intersectionality. *Gender, Place and Culture: A Journal of Feminist Geography*, 22(3), 383–389.

Passaro, J. (2014). *The unequal homeless: Men on the streets, women in their place.* New York, NY: Routledge.

Pease, B. (2010). *Undoing privilege: Unearned advantage in a divided world.* London: Zed Books.

Pease, B. and Flood, M. (2008). Rethinking the significance of attitudes in preventing men's violence against women. *Australian Journal of Social Issues*, 43, 547–561.

Perry, B. (2002). Childhood experience and the expression of genetic potential: What childhood neglect tells us about nature and nurture. *Brain and Mind*, 3, 79–100.

Petriwskyj, A., Gibson, A. and Webby, G. (2015). Staff members' negotiation of power in client engagement: Analysis of practice within an Australian aged care service. *Journal of Aging Studies*, 33, 37–46.

Pilkey, B. (2013a). Queering heteronormativity at home: Older gay Londoners and the negotiation of domestic materiality. *Gender, Place and Culture: A Journal of Feminist Geography*, 21(9), 1142–1157.

Pilkey, B. (2013b). Embodiment of mobile homemaking imaginaries. *Geographical Research*, 51(2), 159–165.

Rowntree, M. (2014). Making sexuality visible in Australian social work education. *Social Work Education*, 33(3), 353–364.

Rowntree, M. and Zufferey, C. (2015). Need or right: Sexual expression and intimacy in aged care. *Journal of Aging Studies*, 35, 20–25.

Smith, A. (2005). Native American feminism, sovereignty, and social change. *Feminist Studies*, 31, 116–132.

Snow, D.A. and Anderson, L. (1987). Identity work among the homeless: The verbal construction and avowal of personal identities. *American Journal of Sociology*, 92, 1336–1371.

Snow, D.A. and Anderson, L. (1993). *Down on their luck: A study of homeless street people.* Berkeley, CA: University of California Press.

Snow, D.A., Leufgen, J. and Cardinale, M. (2007). Homelessness. In G. Ritzer (Ed.). *Blackwell encyclopaedia of sociology.* Blackwell. Accessed 25 February 2014. www.sociologyencyclopedia.com/.

Thomas, L. (2007). *'Are we there yet?' An exploration of the key principles for working with children accessing transitional supported accommodation services.* Canberra, ACT: University of Canberra.

Varney, D. and van Vliet, W. (2008). Homelessness, children, and youth: Research in the United States and Canada. *American Behavioral Scientist*, 51, 715–720.

Walter, M., Taylor, S. and Habibis, D. (2011). How white is social work in Australia? *Australian Social Work*, 64(1), 6–19.

Wasserman, J. and Clair, J. (2010). *At home on the street: People, poverty, and a hidden culture of homelessness.* Boulder, CO: Lynne Rienner.

Watson, J. (2011). Understanding survival sex: Young women, homelessness and intimate relationships. Journal of Youth Studies, 14(6), 639–655.

Yeatman, A. (Ed.). (1998). *Activism and the policy process.* Sydney: Allen and Unwin.

Young, R. (2003). *Postcolonialism: A very short introduction.* Oxford, UK: Oxford University Press.

Zufferey, C. (2001). *Identity and everyday experiences of homelessness: Personal stories from Aboriginal and Non Aboriginal men and women*, MSW Thesis. School of Social Work and Social Policy, University of South Australia.

Zufferey, C. (2013). 'Not knowing that I do not know and not wanting to know': Reflections of a white Australian social worker. *International Social Work*, 56(5), 659–673.

Zufferey, C. (2014). Questioning representations of homelessness in the Australian print media. *Australian Social Work*, 67(4), 525–536.

Zufferey, C. (2015). Diverse meanings of home in multicultural Australia. *The International Journal of Diverse Identities*, 13(2), 13–21.

Zufferey, C. and Chung, D. (2015). Red dust homelessness: Housing, home and homelessness in remote Australia. *Journal of Rural Studies*, 41, 13–22.

Zufferey, C. and Kerr, L. (2004). Identity and everyday experiences of homelessness: Some implications for social work. *Australian Social Work*, 57(4), 343–353

Zufferey, C. and Rowntree, M. (2014). Finding your community wherever you go? Exploring how a group of women who identify as lesbian embody and imagine 'home'. The Australian Sociological Association (TASA) Conference, University of South Australia, 24–27 November, Adelaide.

Zufferey, C., Chung, D., Franzway, S., Wendt, S. and Moulding, N. (2016). Intimate partner violence and housing: Eroding women's citizenship. *Affilia: Journal of Women and Social Work*. DOI: 10.1177/088610991562621.

7 Conclusion

The interrelationships between intersectionality, homelessness and social work are complicated and contested, as is the very notion of intersectionality itself (McKibbin *et al.*, 2015). In this book I have argued that intersectionality is a new way of thinking and theorising about homelessness and social work. I have sought to contribute to social work knowledge by considering an intersectional social work approach to homelessness. This has been achieved by exploring literature and research on intersectionality, social work research, homelessness policy making, practitioner responses and service user perspectives By reflecting on my own Australian social work practice and research on homelessness spanning over two decades, I have illustrated diverse perspectives on home, service providers' responses and service users' experiences of homelessness.

The introductory chapter introduced the main concepts and arguments covered in this book, highlighting that intersecting power relations constitute social work research, social policy and practice responses to homelessness. In Chapter 2, intersectionality was explored in more depth from multiple perspectives using multidisciplinary literature. Chapter 3 examined how intersectionality has (or has not) been used in social work and homelessness research, highlighting numerous gaps in social work literature. I also analysed multidisciplinary literature and presented my own research on home, homelessness (and related areas such as domestic violence) and intersectionality. In Chapter 4 intersectional policy analysis approaches in multidisciplinary literature were outlined. Definitions of homelessness, legislation and service initiatives such as 'Housing First' in the USA, UK, Australia and the European Union were examined, using intersectional policy analysis questions. Chapter 5 discussed and reflected on social work practice responses to homelessness, using literature and research data from interviews with social workers in the field of homelessness, my reflexive commentary and a case study. In this chapter I advocated for social worker self-reflexivity and argued that social work responses to homelessness can be expanded through an intersectional social work approach. Such an approach would enable social workers to gain further insights into how they can promote practices aligned with their commitments to challenging social injustice and human rights violations

(Murphy *et al.*, 2009). Chapter 6 highlighted the diversity of homelessness by documenting research on the 'voices' and experiences of service users and people affected by homelessness. I emphasised the intersectional complexities in people's lives, in the context of experiencing homelessness, by exploring at least two or more 'categories of oppression' (Hulko, 2015, p. 71). In this book I have argued that an intersectional social work approach can provide new ways of moving forward, by incorporating inclusive and participatory service user-led research, to inform social work policy and practice in the area of homelessness.

The contents of this book are consistent with the aims of intersectionality. I acknowledged and centred the voices of people most affected by homelessness (Hulko, 2015); made visible intersecting diversities (Dhamoon, 2011) in the area of homelessness; was 'majority inclusive' by examining social workers' own privileges (Christensen and Jensen, 2012); explored the complexities of oppressive and privileging processes (and identities) in literature (Lykke, 2010); demonstrated how social inequalities and injustices that contribute to homelessness manifest in interconnected domains of power relations (Thornton Dill and Zambrana, 2009; Thornton Dill and Kohlman, 2012); and promoted social justice and social change consistent with the ethics of social work (Murphy *et al.*, 2009). I have struggled with having to limit the scope of this book to focusing only on some intersections, particularly gender, ethnicity/race, sexuality, class and age, which resonate with critiques of intersectionality itself. However, I have argued that the complexities of this book distinguish it from other work in the fields of social work and homelessness.

A new social work approach?

The intersectional social work approach that I have proposed is consistent with social work ethics and values about social change, and working to upholding social justice and human rights (Murphy *et al.*, 2009). There are debates, though, in the field of intersectionality, being led by US and European scholars, about the relative merits of constructionist or systemic approaches to intersectionality (Prins, 2006, p. 277). As outlined in Chapter 2, I have acknowledged ontological differences in the conceptualisation of intersectionality between systemic, structural and post-constructionist/post-structural theorising. I have argued that diverse intersectional approaches, including McCall's (2005) anti-categorical, intra-categorical and inter-categorical dimensions, and Lykke's (2010) more social constructionist approach, can contribute to widening understandings of homelessness and social work responses to it. I have suggested that different intersectional approaches can be relevant to social work and homelessness, depending on the purpose of the research project, policy or practice intervention.

My intersectional social work approach has transcended previous literature in homelessness that examined dynamic interactions between macro structures (such as changes to housing and labour markets), and the micro processes that increase an individual's vulnerability to homelessness. The intersectional approach in this book broadened structural and individual concerns, to focus on how multiple power relations intersect, to both privilege and oppress individuals and community groups differently. This approach can enable social workers to highlight simplistic, homogenous constructions of homelessness that limit how homelessness is thought about. My conceptualisation of intersectionality has aligned with understandings in literature that unequal power relations are influenced by intersecting social structures, organisations and social institutions, as well as cultural and discursive representations of social problems (Winker and Degele, 2011). I also drew on poststructuralist ontologies to explore homeless and social work subjectivities, as being an effect of the power of language and discourse (McKibbin *et al.*, 2015, p. 101).

This intersectional social work approach has promoted reflexivity, which involved reflecting on my own positions and social locations, personally and professionally, as an academic, researcher and practitioner. The social justice assumptions that underpin intersectionality make it particularly useful for examining social work research, policy, practice and education (Murphy *et al.*, 2009). As the production of knowledge in academia has been contained within normative, predominantly white, masculine and middle-class institutionalised discourses and structures (Thornton-Dill and Kohlman, 2012), this has raised questions about whose values, traditions, practices and knowledges are being privileged in the teaching of social work (Roberts and Smith, 2002; Holtzhausen, 2011). These dilemmas are made visible through a reflexive, intersectional analysis of social work responses to homelessness.

Throughout this book I argued that intersectionality is a concept and an approach that is malleable and flexible enough to adapt to the increasingly diversifying 'new' demographics of homelessness across the USA, UK, Australia and the EU. The approach extends social work (and other professionals') understandings about the depth and breadth of the historical, social, political and cultural experiences of our client groups (Murphy *et al.*, 2009, p. 1). Aligned with Murphy *et al.* (2009, p. 87), I argued that intersectionality is a paradigm shift for social work, by focusing on how social inequalities can be maintained through oppressive and privileging practices, within complex contexts and shifting local and global demographics and dynamics particularly pertinent in the changing field of homelessness. Therefore, I also noted that homelessness and social work responses to it have shifted over time and can be reinterpreted in different local and global contexts.

In this book I intended to move beyond focusing on 'individualized politics' (Nixon and Humphreys, 2010), and interrelating identity categories, to exploring how social work responses to homelessness are processes that are socially located. As such, my intersectional approach interrogated social work research, analysed policy-making processes, reflected on social worker's diverse social locations and unpacked client-worker power relations, by exploring lived experiences. This approach and analysis contributed to making visible intersecting social inequalities and provided areas for future social work research and advocacy. I have argued that central to social work's mission for social justice and social change is the questioning of representations of social problems in institutionalised social processes, such as research and policy making, which involves emphasising how inequalities intersect.

Social work research

As outlined in Chapter 3, I found that there was a dearth of social work research literature on homelessness and intersectionality. I posited that an intersectional approach complicated social work and homelessness research, by enabling us to focus on the heterogeneity of people's lives, including the lives of 'homeless people' and social workers, without disregarding the material reality of homelessness. By employing Winker and Degele's (2011) multilayered intersectional analysis, I noted that social workers can research the relationships between social structures, constructions of identities and symbolic representations of social issues. However, social work research, policy and practice are often constructed in relation to symbolic public representations of social work and homelessness, such as in the media. This was evident when I examined print media representations of homelessness that framed constructions of homelessness as a social problem to be 'fixed' by service providers such as social workers (Zufferey, 2014). Media coverage of social issues such as homelessness has tended to fix homeless and housed identities (Hodgetts *et al.*, 2006, p. 498), and construct simplistic solutions to the issue. The intersectional social work approach has challenged simplistic policy responses to and media representations of homelessness and social work.

This book illustrated how social work research, policy and practice are diverse, with multiple understandings of and responses to homelessness. Consistent with Hulko's (2015) research, I have adopted an intersectional approach to social work research, and contributed to promoting new research paradigms and practices that involved being reflexive, collaborative and participatory, sampling for diversity, asking questions about (intersecting) social locations, facilitating voice, such as through creative use of methods (such as using visual artefacts, see Zufferey and Rowntree, 2014), and disseminating findings with a view to social change.

Social work policy

As outlined in Chapter 4, I examined the complexities of policy making by using intersectional policy analysis frameworks such as Hankivsky's (2012) Intersectionality-Based Policy Analysis (IBPA). Another particularly useful policy analysis framework was Bacchi's (2009) 'What's the problem represented to be?' (WPR). This policy analysis framework provided a new and different approach to analysing how 'governing' takes place, through questioning the solutions proposed to social problems (such as homelessness) in policy documents, drawing out implications for those who are 'governed' (Bacchi, 2009, p. vii). Drawing on the WPR framework, I have previously examined print media discourses of homelessness (Zufferey, 2014). Intersectionality-Based Policy Analysis (IBPA) partly incorporates Bacchi's WPR approach and has been used for analysing health and public policy (Hankivsky *et al.*, 2014). I argued that the IBPA can also provide for a new way of analysing homelessness policies by exploring whether a policy has transformed thinking about 'relations and structures of power and inequity' (Hankivsky, 2012, pp. 40–42). When I examined definitions of homelessness and statutory legislation in the USA, UK, Australia and Europe, as well as Housing First initiatives, I found that legislation and policies have partly transformed social work thinking about homelessness but have failed to intersect multiple social discriminations. Future areas for policy advocacy were identified, which included incorporating diverse understandings of homelessness that move beyond housing-based policy definitions of homelessness (Zufferey and Chung, 2015).

I have argued that an intersectional approach to policy making addresses intersecting power relations, discriminatory practices and social inequalities contributing to homelessness. This approach expands on current homelessness advocacy that makes visible: few housing options, the lack of accessible and safe housing, limited access to services such as income security, employment, education and health care, and recognising [homeless people's] right to be recognised 'as citizens of dignity and worth equal to that of other citizens' (Coleman, 2012, p. 278). This advocacy has included focusing on the individual-structural dynamics of homelessness (Johnson *et al.*, 2015). In this book, I have argued that an intersectional policy approach (Parken, 2010; Hankivsky and Cormier, 2011) to homelessness incorporates *intersecting* diversities and inequalities, while promoting human rights initiatives in social policy, which broadens theorising about macro (structural) as well as micro (everyday) social change.

Social work practice

In Chapter 5, I contended that an intersectional social work approach provides new possibilities for reflecting on and responding to homelessness. Social work is socially located and positioned within organisational contexts and social institutions that are unequal, multilayered, dynamic and complex. Within these social and organisational contexts, social workers embody institutionalised gendered, classed, heteronormative and racialised practices. I have argued that intersectional approaches invite social workers to engage in reflexive practices that acknowledge their own intersecting privileges (and oppressions) and embodied subjectivities. Further, by attending to intersecting social inequalities that contribute to homelessness, social workers can complement the actions of differently positioned advocates for homelessness (such as service users), creating possibilities for 'coalitional activism and social change' (Jones, 2010, p. 122).

My argument is that social workers are involved in maintaining social inequalities because they are often employed in organisations and social institutions that have institutionalised heteronormative, gendered, classed, racialised and xenophobic practices. However, they are also involved in resisting discriminatory practices and advocating for social change. That is, social workers can be involved in constructing as well as challenging 'one size fits all' policy and practice responses to homelessness, that are often criticised by people who experience homelessness, for not being diverse, inclusive and heterogeneous enough (Zufferey and Kerr, 2004). I posited that an intersectional analysis can deconstruct and make visible social work practices and processes that contribute to maintaining (and resisting) intersecting social inequalities. This exploration can also highlight the diverse effects of social work practices on people who experience homelessness. Overall, I have argued that an intersectional approach can contribute to social workers advocating for new ways of thinking about social work research, policy and practice in the field of homelessness.

Summary

In summary, homelessness and social work in different countries are influenced by differing legislation, political systems, welfare states, understandings of social work and homelessness. This book cannot cover all background contexts, areas and countries. I have limited the discussion to examining social work and research trends in homelessness in the contexts of noteworthy literature from Australia, UK, Canada, USA and the European Union. Below I list what I see as the key points when considering an intersectional social work approach in the field of homelessness in these Western contexts:

1   Social workers themselves are not exempt from the subjectifying practices and intersecting inequalities that function to continue to oppress and also privilege certain members of society. However, intersecting influences that oppress or privilege are contextual and dynamic in their effects and continue to shift and change over time and place.
2   Historical social work practices and homogenous constructions of 'the homeless experience' cannot be ignored when examining how intersecting inequalities influence a socially constructed problem such as homelessness. However, whilst sexism, racism, classism, heterosexism and 'third worldism' continue to exist and produce unequal power relations, the effects of these on human experiences constantly change and are constituted through different political, social, economic and cultural contexts.
3   Diverse perspectives on intersectionality are inevitable and provide for its flexibility. Different 'ways of doing' intersectionality can be incorporated into social work research designs and paradigms, multiple levels of social work practice (such as micro, mezzo and macro) and social policy development and analysis. An intersectional social work approach is more inclusive of the complexity and diversity of homelessness, compared to

traditional social work approaches that tend to privilege one pre-selected social inequality (such as class, gender or race), and 'silo' responses in social work research, social policy and 'frontline' practice.

4   Material experiences and social constructions of Indigeneity, race, class, gender, age, sexuality, (dis)ability, nationalism, social and geographical locations intersect to constitute the subjectivities of both social workers and service users (including people who experience homelessness). These institutionalised material practices, discursive representations and social constructions have implications for how social workers understand and respond to homelessness in research, policy and practice. However, given that the social work profession has a commitment to influencing social change and promoting social justice, an intersectional social work approach would include challenging discriminatory processes and intersecting social inequalities that disadvantage particular population groups, such as people who experience homelessness.

This book has acknowledged that social work responses to homelessness are historically and socially constructed within, for example, intersecting classed, gendered and racialised processes. Social work research, policy and practice are influenced by social worker's own intersecting social locations, and the social work profession itself is affected by being predominantly white, middle-class, heteronormative and gendered. Furthermore, social work has been constructed within particular historical values about class, gender, family, work, age and sexuality (Abrams, 2000; Cree, 2002, p. 280) that continue to influence contemporary practices. In this book, I have argued for an intersectional social work approach that can make visible intersecting power relations that shape the subjectivities of people who experience homelessness, as well as the social work research, policy and practice processes. By attending carefully to these processes, I have argued that an intersectional social work approach can enable social workers to broaden their critical analysis and advocacy responses to homelessness. However, I would also like to acknowledge that an intersectional social work approach can be applied to other fields of research, policy and practice, besides homelessness. My hope for the future is that this intersectional social work approach can be further developed and expanded on by other scholars, to contribute to future possibilities for social work, that extend within and beyond the profession.

References

Abrams, L.S. (2000). Guardians of virtue: The social reformers and the 'girl problem', 1890–1920. *Social Services Review*, 74(3), 436–452.

Bacchi, C. (2009). *Analysing policy: What's the problem represented to be?* Sydney: Pearson.

Christensen, A. and Jensen, S. (2012). Doing intersectional analysis: Methodological implications for qualitative research. *Nordic Journal of Feminist and Gender Research*, 20(2), 109–125.

Coleman, A. (2012). Context, context, context: A commentary on responding to people sleeping rough: Dilemmas and opportunities for social work (Parsell, 2011). *Australian Social Work*, 65(2), 274–279.

Cree, V.E. (2002). *Social work and society*. (pp. 275–287). In M. Davies (Ed.). *Blackwell companion to social work* (2nd ed.). Oxford, UK: Blackwell.

Dhamoon, R. (2011). Considerations on mainstreaming intersectionality. *Political Research Quarterly*, 64(1), 230–243.

Hankivsky, O. (Ed.). (2012). *An intersectionality-based policy analysis framework*. Vancouver, BC: Institute for Intersectionality Research and Policy, Simon Fraser University.

Hankivsky, O. and Cormier, R. (2011). Intersectionality and public policy: Some lessons from existing models. *Political Research Quarterly*, 64(1), 217–229.

Hankivsky, O., Grace, D., Hunting, G., Giesbrecht, M., Fridkin, A., Rudrum, S., Ferlatte, O. and Clark, N. (2014). An intersectionality-based policy analysis framework: Critical reflections on a methodology for advancing equity. *International Journal for Equity in Health*, 13(119). Accessed 4 May 2016. DOI: 10.1186/s12939-014-0119-x.

Hodgetts, D., Hodgetts, A. and Radley, A. (2006). Life in the shadow of the media: Imaging street homelessness in London. *European Journal of Cultural Studies*, 9, 497–516.

Holtzhausen, L. (2011). When values collide: Finding common ground for social work education in the United Arab Emirates. *International Social Work*, 54(2), 191–208.

Hulko, W. (2015). Operationalizing intersectionality in feminist social work research: Reflections and techniques from research with equity-seeking groups. (pp. 69–89). In S. Wahab, B. Anderson-Nathe and C. Gringeri (Eds). *Feminisms in social work research*. New York, NY: Routledge.

Johnson, G., Scutella, R., Tseng, Y. and Wood, G. (2015). *Entries and exits from homelessness: A dynamic analysis of the relationship between structural conditions and individual characteristics*. AHURI Final Report No. 248. Melbourne, Vic: Australian Housing and Urban Research Institute. Accessed 12 May 2016. www.ahuri.edu.au/publications/projects/p53042.

Jones, R.G. (2010). Putting privilege into practice through 'intersectional reflexivity': Ruminations, interventions, and possibilities. *Faculty Research and Creative Activity*. Paper 3. Accessed 12 May 2016. http://thekeep.eiu.edu/commstudies_fac/3.

Lykke, N. (2010). *Feminist studies: A guide to intersectional theory, methodology, and writing*. New York, NY: Routledge.

McCall, L. (2005). The complexity of intersectionality. *Signs: Journal of Women in Culture and Society*, 30(3), 1771–1800.

McKibbin, G., Duncan, R., Hamilton, B., Cathy Humphreys, C. and Kellett, C. (2015). The intersectional turn in feminist theory: A response to Carbin and Edenheim (2013). *European Journal of Women's Studies*, 22(1), 99–103.

Murphy, Y., Hunt, V., Zajicek, A.M., Norris, A.N. and Hamilton, L. (2009). *Incorporating intersectionality in social work practice, research, policy, and education*. Washington, DC: NASW Press.

Nixon, J. and Humphreys, C. (2010). Marshalling the evidence: Using intersectionality in the domestic violence frame. *Social Politics*, 17(2), 137–158.

Parken, A. (2010). A multi-strand approach to promoting equality and human rights in policymaking. *Policy and Politics*, 38(1), 79–99.

Prins, B. (2006). Narrative accounts of origins: A blind spot in the intersectional approach. *European Journal of Women's Studies. Special Issue on Intersectionality*, 13(3), 277–290.

Roberts, T.L. and Smith, L.A. (2002). The illusion of inclusion: An analysis of approaches to diversity within predominantly white schools of social work. *Journal of Teaching in Social Work*, 22(3), 189–211.

Thornton Dill, B. and Kohlman, M.H. (2012). Intersectionality. (pp. 154–171). In S. Hesse-Biber (Ed.). *Handbook of feminist research*. Los Angeles, CA: Sage.

Thornton Dill, B. and Zambrana, R.E. (2009). *Emerging intersections: Race, class, and gender in theory, policy, and practice*. Piscataway, NJ: Rutgers University Press.

Winker, G. and Degele, N. (2011). Intersectionality as multi-level analysis: Dealing with social inequality. *European Journal of Women's Studies*, 18(1), 51–66.

Zufferey, C. (2014). Questioning representations of homelessness in the Australian print media. *Australian Social Work*, 67(4), 525–536.

Zufferey, C. and Chung, D. (2015). 'Red dust homelessness': housing, home and homelessness in remote Australia. *Journal of Rural Studies*, 41, 13–22.

Zufferey, C. and Kerr, L. (2004). Identity and everyday experiences of homelessness: Some implications for social work. *Australian Social Work*, 57(4), 343–353.

Zufferey, C. and Rowntree, M. (2014). *Finding your community wherever you go? Exploring how a group of women who identify as lesbian embody and imagine 'home'*. The Australian Sociological Association (TASA) Conference, University of South Australia, 24–27 November, Adelaide.

Index